Praise for *Beyond the Blues*

"Shoshana and Pec have designed an easy-to-use format for all practitioners who work with childbearing women. While the topic is extremely complex, their book provides the most essential information in a concise manner. This is a long overdue contribution to the field of maternal mental health. Thank you Shoshana and Pec!"

—**Jane Honikman, MS, Founder**
Postpartum Support International

"In *Beyond the Blues*, Bennett and Indman offer a compact yet surprisingly comprehensive manual on prenatal and postpartum depression. Readable and practical, they systematically address screening and assessment, finding a therapist, myths about nursing and bonding, and treatment. Interesting and helpful are suggestions for family and friends. For health professionals, there is detailed diagnostic and treatment information. *Beyond the Blues* is a quick read with an easy-to-handle format. Recommended for consumer health and health sciences collections."

—*Library Journal*

"As a nonprofit advocate and leader, my go-to book about maternal mental health disorders is *Beyond the Blues*. We promote the book through our work with hospitals, insurers, clinicians and advocates. Our followers find the book is a page-turner and provides just the right amount of information about maternal mental health disorders."

—**Joy Burkhard, MBA**
Founder and Director, Policy Center for Maternal Mental
Health

"I love this book! It is easy to read and use as an informative reference for all aspects of perinatal mood and anxiety disorders. I recommend this book to all the OB care provider offices in my hospital system. It's an excellent book for my clients and required reading for providers I train. Thanks to Pec and Shoshana for the recent updates which make this great book even better."

—**Birdie Gunyon Meyer, RN, MA**
Indiana Coordinator, Postpartum Support International
Past President, Postpartum Support International

"Refreshingly easy to read and understand. Informative, concise and truly user friendly. A valuable tool for clinicians and consumers alike."

—**Joyce A. Venis, RNC, Past President**
Depression After Delivery, Inc.
Director of Nursing, Princeton Family Care Associates

"Succinct yet informative, a useful guide for the busy practitioner or overwhelmed mother."

—**Valerie Raskin, MD, Psychiatrist**
Author of *This Isn't What I Expected* and
When Words Are Not Enough

"I lost my wife, Kristin Brooks Rossell, to suicide following a four-month battle with postpartum psychosis. All the things one should not do in the treatment of this deadly disease were done to Kristin. *Beyond the Blues* is a step-by-step guide that would have saved her life. *Beyond the Blues* is not long, yet its content is comprehensive and well written. I cried reading each page, knowing at each turn how this information could have been used to save Kristin, myself, and our families the pain and needless suffering we experienced."

—**H. Reese Butler II**

"An indispensable guide to understanding and treating prenatal and postpartum depression. This book is a gift not only to healthcare providers but also to family and friends of mothers suffering from these devastating perinatal mood disorders."

—Cheryl Tatano Beck, DNSc, CNM, FAAN Professor
University of Connecticut, School of Nursing
Coauthor of *Postpartum Depression Screening Scale*

"After reading *Beyond the Blues*, I immediately ordered several copies and shared them with colleagues. It is a wonderful resource, easy to read and full of practical wisdom. I've worked with postpartum families for many years and learned a great deal reading this book."

—Maggie Muir, LMFT, IBCLC, Nursing Mothers Counsel

"As a psychotherapist treating postpartum women, I have referred to the information in this book over and over. Drs. Indman and Bennett are two reliable sources who have checked all their facts while intelligently turning this very complex topic into something so clear and understandable."

—Kim Richardson, MA, LCPC

"Provides practical, easy-to-follow advice for moms, dads, grandparents, and more. Most importantly, Shoshana and Pec paint a clear picture of this horrible illness. They provided me with a constant reminder that my wife was not alone in her suffering and would absolutely recover with proper care. The book provided hope at a time when it was hard to find."

—Mark S.

"*Beyond the Blues* by Shoshana Bennett and Pec Indman is a very insightful, concise, informative manual that should be in the hands of all providers and new mothers dealing with postpartum depression. It is a fantastic book containing all the necessary questions and answers."

—**Shirley Halvorson, Past President, Depression After Delivery (North Carolina), Past Coordinator, Postpartum Support International (North Carolina)**

"This valuable treatment manual should be in the pocket of every practitioner who works with women. It is well researched and indexed for quick and easy reference by healthcare providers as well as clients and their families. As a registered nurse and lactation consultant, I have found it invaluable in assisting new mothers to comfortably achieve the breastfeeding experience they want with their babies. Thanks for dispelling so many of the old myths!"

—**Pat Ross, RN, IBCLC, Kaiser Permanente**

"Before I read this book I thought I was the only mother who felt this way. It was reassuring to know that I wasn't alone! My husband read the chapter for partners and he finally knew what to say to help me."

—**Patty B.**

"This book is an invaluable guide not only for women experiencing these disorders, but should also be mandatory reading for all who work with women during pregnancy and postpartum. It is a true breakthrough on the topic of prenatal and postpartum depression. This is the one book you should have on your shelf."

—Lisa Nakamura, Postpartum Doula
Nurturing Mother Postpartum Services

"I never knew you could be depressed when you're pregnant. I was told that the pregnancy hormones would keep the depression away. I was severely depressed two months ago and my mother found *Beyond the Blues* for me. Now I am eight months pregnant, and I can't wait for my baby!"

—Carole B.

"I didn't know what to do when my wife started crying all the time after we came home from the hospital. The obstetrician handed me this book and finally things started making sense. It wasn't easy, but we made it through. The chapter for husbands was really useful for me because it told me what I should and shouldn't do to help my wife."

—Jeff B.

"*Beyond the Blues* is an informative and educational tool for ALL interested in gaining or enhancing their knowledge of prenatal and postpartum depression. Its simplified and direct approach is truly appreciated. As a mom and clinical social worker, I highly recommend this book. As a matter of fact, I already do!"

—Joy Fullhardt, LCSW, ACSW

Beyond the Blues

*Understanding and Treating
Prenatal and Postpartum
Depression & Anxiety*

Shoshana S. Bennett, PhD, PMH-C
Pec Indman, PA, EdD, MFT, PMH-C

Beyond the Blues

*Understanding and Treating
Prenatal and Postpartum
Depression & Anxiety*

6th Edition
Revised and Updated

Histria Perspectives

Las Vegas ♦ Chicago ♦ Palm Beach

Published in the United States of America by Histria Books
7181 N. Hualapai Way, Ste. 130-86
Las Vegas, NV 89166 U.S.A.
HistriaBooks.com

Histria Perspectives is an imprint of Histria Books and a joint venture of Histria Books and Creative Destruction Media. Titles published under the imprints of Histria Books are distributed worldwide.

Library of Congress Control Number: 2024940858

ISBN 978-1-59211-528-0 (hardcover)
ISBN 978-1-59211-533-4 (softbound)
ISBN 978-1-59211-541-9 (eBook)

This Book is Dedicated to

Our children Elana, Aaron, Megan, and Emily
for teaching us about being moms.
And to our dear clients,
who trust us with their deepest fears and greatest hopes.

Acknowledgments

We want to thank K.D. Sullivan at Histria Books, and express our appreciation to all who contributed to this book. We are grateful to our wonderful research colleagues who help us better understand, prevent, and treat perinatal mood and anxiety disorders. Throughout the text we have referenced some of their valuable work and you will find the complete citations in the Resources section. The authors gratefully acknowledge the research assistance provided by Mike Liddicoat, Senior Medical Librarian at El Camino Health.

Shoshana S. Bennett, PhD, PMH-C
DrShosh.com

Pec Indman, PA, EdD, MFT, PMH-C
Pecfish@gmail.com

Contents

Foreword v

Preface vii

Introduction ix

One: Our Stories 1

    Shoshana's Story 1

    Pec's Story 8

Two: Perinatal Psychiatric Illness 11

    Perinatal Mood and Anxiety Disorders 13

    The Psychiatric Issues of Pregnancy 14

    Depression and Anxiety in Pregnancy 15

    After the Birth, "Baby Blues"—Not a Disorder 18

    Depression and Anxiety Postpartum 19

    Obsessive-Compulsive Disorder (OCD) 22

    Panic Disorder 24

    Psychosis 26

    Post-traumatic Stress Disorder (PTSD) 27

    Bipolar Disorder I or II (sometimes referred to as Bipolar Spectrum Disorder) 29

    Consequences of *Untreated* Depression in Parents 30

    Perinatal Loss 32

Three: Perinatal Disorders 33

    Finding a Therapist or Medical Practitioner 34

    The Truth of the Matter 35

    Basic Mom Care 36

    Myths About Using Breast Milk 44

    Recovery 47

    Antidepressant Questions and Answers 47

Four: Partners 53

    Things to Keep in Mind 55

    What to Say, What Not to Say 57

    From a Dad Who's Been There 59

Five: Family and Friends 61

Communicating with Children 62

Things to Keep in Mind 64

What to Say, What Not to Say 65

What You Can Do to Help 66

Six: Practitioners **69**

Culture and Language 70

What to Say, What Not to Say 71

Screening 72

Prenatal Screening 73

Pre-pregnancy and Pregnancy Risk Assessment 73

Postpartum Screening 76

Postpartum Risk Assessment 77

Psychotherapists, Psychologists, Social Workers 80

Primary Care Providers 80

Pediatricians and Neonatologists 81

OB/GYNs, Midwives, and Other Women's Healthcare Providers 82

Psychiatrists and Other Psychiatric Prescribers 83

Birth Doulas 83

Postpartum Doulas , Visiting Nurses, and Home Visitors 84

Lactation Consultants 85

Childbirth Educators 86

New Parent Group Leaders 87

Adjunct Professionals 88

Seven: Treatment **89**

Why Is Treatment Necessary? 89

When Dads Have Depression 90

Research 91

Prevention 92

Psychotherapy 94

Social Support 96

Complementary and Alternative Medicine (CAM) 96

Medications for PMADs 102

Pregnancy and Medication 103

Antianxiety Medications 104

Postpartum 111

Medications and Breast Milk 113
Medical Protocols 115

Resources **119**
Websites and Helplines 119
Journal Articles 122

Appendix **151**
Terminology 151
Healthcare Professionals 157

Endorsements and Awards **161**

Seminars, Training, Workshops, and Consultation **163**

About the Authors **165**

Index **167**

Foreword

This fine publication fills the education void between sufferers of postpartum disorders (women, men, and families) and healthcare professionals. Concise information is provided for all! Those of us who do clinical work and research in perinatal psychiatry define therapies, evaluate effects of medication for breastfeeding babies, explore preventive treatment, and much more—all very important endeavors. But the community of parents must be connected to well-informed professionals in order for even the most exciting of data to be put to use.

A very warm thank you to these two dedicated women for their commitment and sensitivity, and to Shoshana and Henry for their willingness to share the pain of their postpartum experience. It is my sincere hope that the countless people who read this book will benefit from your pain, thereby lessening the intensity of its memory.

Katherine L. Wisner, MD, MS

Norman and Helen Asher Professor of Psychiatry
and Behavioral Sciences and Obstetrics and Gynecology

Director, Asher Center for the Study
and Treatment of Depressive Disorders

Feinberg School of Medicine,
Department of Psychiatry and Behavioral Sciences,
Northwestern University

Preface

Prenatal and postpartum mood and anxiety disorders are very common. In the United States alone, over 3.7 million women give birth each year. Since the rate of perinatal (pregnancy through the first postpartum year) depression is about 20%, at least 740,000 of these women will become ill.

The rate of gestational diabetes is between 1% and 3%, and the rate of a baby with Down syndrome occurring in a 35-year-old mother is 3%. Curiously, screening is routine for these conditions, yet screening for perinatal mental health illnesses—which occur in 1 in 5 mothers—is not.

While working in our communities, we have been asked numerous times to provide simple guidelines for assessment and treatment of perinatal mood and anxiety disorders. Mothers and their partners have been asking the question, "Why is this happening to us and what can we do about it?" Many good books and journal articles have already been written on this topic. Our main goal is to summarize the most current research and information into a practical, easy-to-use format.

This book is not meant to be used as a replacement for individual counseling, group support, or medical assessment, nor do we intend it to be a comprehensive textbook. *Beyond the Blues* will provide critical information for providers and families. Our intention is to offer the most essential and up-to-date assessment, treatment, and resources possible. In the

Appendix you will find definitions of the terms used throughout the book.

While we attempt to be inclusive, we want to acknowledge that almost all of the research has focused on birth mothers or fathers. It's our hope that research will extend in the future to the wide variety of families who raise children, including grandparents.

Introduction

Welcoming a new baby is like opening one of life's big doors of possibilities. Anything can happen. As healthcare providers we do our best to help parents prepare for the birth, yet often gloss over the reality that bringing home a newborn with its own temperament and round-the-clock feeding will undoubtedly lead to a major life adjustment.

A mother must recover from her birth experience while her body undergoes a tremendous hormonal upheaval that rivals any roller coaster ride. Sleep deprivation alone can leave her stumbling around the house in a fog. She is also getting to know her newborn while confronting the loss of her previous life and any sense of control over her time.

Can this be overwhelming and lead to perinatal mental health problems? The answer is yes, and yet it's not hopeless. Perinatal mood and anxiety disorders are conditions that will go away with excellent help. Women, partners, and families do recover and are able to enjoy their lives fully. *Beyond the Blues, Understanding and Treating Prenatal and Postpartum Depression & Anxiety* is a resource that has helped countless healthcare providers, parents, and families to recognize the signs of perinatal illness and help those who are struggling.

Beyond the Blues is up to date with the most current research. It's easy to understand and offers practical, concise explanations. With a straightforward approach that brings the topic into the light, a range of effective solutions is discussed. *Beyond the Blues* also helps eliminate the stigma and shame that have been associated with perinatal illness. The support and guidance for moms, partners, and families is based on over 55 years of combined experience by the two authors.

Beyond the Blues is an excellent resource for professionals and for those suffering. This book has assisted me in helping new parents when they're struggling. This is clearly the best mental health guide I've ever used in my practice. I'm so convinced of its value, I keep copies in my office to give away to those in need.

—**Barbara Dehn, RN, MS, NP**
("Nurse Barb")

One

Our Stories

We arrived at this professional focus by very different paths, one through personal suffering, the other through social activism.

Shoshana's Story

My husband Henry and I happily awaited the birth of our first child. We enjoyed a wonderful marriage and had planned carefully for the addition of children to our home. We had both grown up in healthy, stable families with solid value systems. We were well-educated people with successful careers: my husband, a human resources professional, and I, a special education teacher. I had worked with children for years, beginning with my first babysitting job at age 10.

I felt quite confident taking care of children. The picture I had of my future always included children of my own. I prided myself on being a self-reliant person, able to manage well even under difficult circumstances. Henry came from a family of five children and had always planned on having a large family. We had many well-thought-out plans for the future, and we looked forward with eager anticipation to being parents.

I felt terrific during pregnancy, both physically and emotionally. After childbirth classes, Henry and I felt prepared for the big event. There was one quick mention of C-sections and no mention at all about possible mood difficulties during pregnancy or after delivery. These classes were all about breathing techniques and what to pack in your hospital bag. On the top of every sheet on the note pad our teacher gave us appeared the words, "No drugs please." And it was also assumed, of course, that every woman would choose to breastfeed.

I endured five and a half days of prodromal labor (real labor, but unproductive), during which I could not sleep due to the discomfort. This was followed by another day of hard labor (still prodromal). My baby was transverse (sideways) and posterior ("sunny side up"), a position that caused severe back labor as well. I writhed as the sledgehammer-like pain hit to the front, then with no break, hit to the back. After I hadn't slept for almost a week, my insides were so sore and exhausted I thought I would literally die. At that moment a very strange thing happened. I suddenly became aware that I was hovering over myself, watching myself in pain. Although at the time I had no words to label that bizarre sensation, I now know it to be called an out-of-body experience. Still not dilating, I was finally given a C-section.

My illusion of being in control was shattered. I had been a professional dancer, and my body had always done what I had wanted it to. The visual image I repeatedly had during this ghastly time was of a beautiful, perfect, clear glass ball violently exploding into millions of pieces. That was the self I felt I was losing. Hopelessness and helplessness replaced my previous feelings of control and independence. I was left with a post-traumatic stress disorder that haunted me for years.

I soon learned a skill that I would practice for a very long time—acting. I bought into the myths that I was supposed to feel instant joy and fulfillment in my role as a mother, as well as an immediate emotional attachment to my baby. As my daughter, Elana, was placed in my arms, I managed to say all my lines correctly. "Hi, honey, I'm so happy you're finally here," I said, wanting to feel it. Inside, I was numb.

Overwhelm, fear, and doom intensified as my first OB appointment approached. While I drove to the doctor's office, my anxiety level rose to unimaginable heights. I pulled my car over to the shoulder of the freeway. Hunched over the steering wheel, I experienced my first panic attack. When I returned home and called to apologize for missing my appointment, I perceived only a tone of annoyance—instead of concern—from the receptionist.

I had lost all the baby weight in the hospital, but just four months postpartum, I was forty pounds overweight. I had always enjoyed a wonderful working relationship with my OB, and felt that he respected me as an intelligent patient. Now, coming to his office as a hand-wringing, depressed mess, I felt embarrassed and vulnerable. As I sat in the waiting room surrounded by mothers-to-be and women cuddling their newborns, my feelings of guilt intensified. I became totally convinced that I should never have become a mother.

Though my OB was well-meaning, his technician-like manner was anything but reassuring. He focused primarily on my incision, not my huge weight gain or uncontrolled crying. With tremendous shame, I confessed some of my feelings to him, including, "If life's going to be like this, I don't want to be here anymore." I was shocked and hurt when he leaned back in his chair, laughed, and said, "This is normal. All moms feel these blues." He gave me his home number so I could call his wife, but he provided no referral. As my ten-minute appointment came to a close, I began to experience my first serious suicidal thoughts.

I did call his wife, who was convinced my problem was that the baby was manipulating me. I just needed to put her on a schedule. I also reluctantly joined a new moms' group; since everyone was suggesting it, I decided to try. That was one of the most destructive actions I took. As I entered the room full of mothers cradling their babies with delight, I felt more alienated than ever.

Discussing "problems" in this group meant pondering the best way to remove formula stains from fabrics, managing spit-up, and calming a fussy baby. When I mentioned that I was having a bad time, an uncomfortable silence fell. I learned later that my name had been removed from the group's babysitting co-op. Upon leaving the first and only group session I attended, I felt more inadequate and scared than ever. Now I knew I was the worst mother that ever walked the planet.

Another complication was breastfeeding. Although my daughter latched on easily, I was overcome with pain due to inflammation and bleeding. I had been one of the "good" students who had prepared her nipples before birth, just as the nurses had suggested—rubbing them with a washcloth to toughen them up. I asked a leader from a prominent lactation organization to help me.

While the representative proved to be very helpful with suggestions about relieving the pains of breastfeeding, her emotional support immediately ended when I divulged that I would be going back to work in six months and would have to discontinue breastfeeding. She abruptly left my home. At this point I made the decision to stop breastfeeding completely, feeling like a total failure.

Life at home was frightening and unbearable. I had full-blown postpartum obsessive-compulsive disorder. Terrifying thoughts of harming my baby plagued me. I could imagine every household item possibly hurting my innocent child. Accidentally tossing my baby over the second-floor railing, dropping her into the fireplace, or putting her in the microwave were common worries. I would not trust myself to be alone with her. Not even my husband knew about these horrible thoughts—I could barely admit them to myself.

If I could sleep at all, I awoke in a full panic attack, wondering if I could survive another day. The simple act of watching television could turn an already dreary day into a deeper depression. The commercials portraying mothers in wavy white dresses with naked babies in their arms, taking delight in changing diapers and smiling angelically at their bundles of joy, sent me further into the depths. These were subtle reminders of the differences between all other mothers and me.

When my husband left for work, I would beg, "Don't leave me, I can't do this by myself!" He would return from work to find me in the same emotional state as when he left. I still remember my husband peering in the front window each night with that worried look, trying to see how many of us were crying. If it was just one, it was I.

Henry was frustrated with me. His mother, who had been a postpartum nurse for 20 years and who had popped out five babies of her own without the least dose of the "blues," was feeding Henry unhelpful information like, "Shoshana is a mother now. She needs to stop complaining and just do it." My respite came each evening as I tossed Henry the baby, proceeded to the driveway, jumped into the car, and sat and cried for a half hour. There was no laughter, no humor, no friends, and no plans. There was only despair.

My mother had come to stay with us for the first three weeks. She was wonderfully supportive, but even with her therapist background she did not recognize the signs of this serious illness. For the next year I continued on my downward spiral. I allowed no emotional or physical connection with my husband. I continued to be deprived of sleep due to insomnia and anxiety, ate without experiencing much taste, and just went through the motions with my daughter. I felt buried alive with no chance of clawing my way to the surface. I saw a psychologist who never once requested any historical data on depression or anxiety in my family. All she did was probe for issues in my past, and if she couldn't find a real one, she would make one up. First she blamed my grandmother, then my sister. Finally she tried to convince me that having a cesarean delivery caused my condition. I ended up feeling "crazier" than I did before I saw her. I swore I would never again open up to another professional. When Elana was 2½ years old, my anxiety and depression began to lift significantly. "Maybe I can be a mother," I heard myself saying. My hair began to curl again for the first time since the birth. I began to enjoy my food, and started seeing in color again, rather than shades of gray.

As with my first pregnancy, my second was flawless and without complication. I was enjoying my daughter by then, and the thought of a second child was a delight. After two days of prodromal labor, I decided on a C-section. The newfound enjoyment and relief from depression came to a crashing halt immediately after the birth of our son, Aaron. Although I could physically take care of him, my former "I'm incompetent" feelings returned. I would easily lose my temper at Elana, who was only 3½ years old. Having been a teacher and knowing child development, I could not find words for my shame and guilt at the way I was treating her. The brief amount of time she had her mom "all there" was suddenly ripped away from her.

In 1987, when Aaron was almost a year old, Henry excitedly called me to look at a television documentary he was watching on postpartum depression. I was awestruck as the program described the disorder, its symptoms, causes, and possible cures. At the program's conclusion, I cried for an hour, looked at my husband, and said, "That's me!" The tremendous sensation of relief that someone had, at long last, described the turbulent agony I had been living felt like a weight being lifted from my whole body. Equally important, I had finally heard that postpartum depression is diagnosable and treatable and that it can go away! If this condition is so common, I thought, where are all of us? And why are we and our families being allowed to suffer without help from professionals?

I started reading everything I could get my hands on, from all over the world, and realized that many countries were light-years ahead of the United States in recognizing and treating postpartum mental health problems. In my research, I came across Jane Honikman in Santa Barbara, founder of Postpartum Support International.

Jane generously offered me valuable information so that I could begin running a self-help group in the San Francisco Bay Area.

Although I was still depressed myself, I was excited about what I had been learning and wanted to share my knowledge with other sufferers and survivors. In contrast to the new-mothers' group I had attended, my group would be a safe place for women to discuss their depression and anxiety openly, without fear of judgment. There was no Internet yet in the 1980s. I posted two flyers, one at a local supermarket, the other at my pediatrician's office. The response was thunderous! Calls came in from all over Northern California and some from as far away as Hawaii. Every week my living room was filled with six to fifteen women, desperate for support and guidance.

I became convinced that postpartum illness needed the same support, psychological attention, and medical tools as other mental illnesses. This began my mission to begin a new career devoted to the study and treatment of postpartum mood and anxiety disorders. Since then I have become a clinical psychologist, founded a local organization, became president of California's state organization Postpartum Health Alliance, and president of Postpartum Support International. I was asked to write three books following *Beyond the Blues*, created the first app for PPD, and am the executive director of the film, *Dark Side of The Full Moon*. Jane Honikman and I cofounded and currently run the Parental Action Institute, and I serve on the President's Advisory Council for Postpartum Support International.

For over 37 years, the support groups which began in my living room have continued and flourished. As a speaker, author, and psychologist I am joyfully continuing to pursue my life's work.

Pec's Story

For as long as I can remember, I have been interested in political, emotional, and sociological issues as they relate to women. In the 1970s I trained as a family practice physician assistant and worked in community-based family health clinics for a number of years. My interests varied, and my work took me to such places as women's clinics, an industry-based employee health center, a physical and fitness evaluation center, and weight-management programs.

I entered a master's program in health psychology and then decided to continue with a doctorate in counseling, receiving my marriage and family therapy (MFT) license along the way. Many of my clients were referred by physicians, and much of my work with clients, particularly women, centered on issues related to health and emotional well-being.

One day, while in a physician's waiting room before a meeting, I came across a brochure from Postpartum Support International that described postpartum depression. I scribbled down the address, thinking, "I need to learn more about this." After receiving more information about PPD, I had a very mixed emotional response. I experienced sadness, extreme anger, frustration, and outrage. In all my years of training, I had learned nothing about perinatal mood disorders. I thought back to some of the women I had probably misdiagnosed. Why aren't health practitioners taught about PPD? My anger propelled me into action.

My second daughter was born when I was forty, after a workup for infertility, a laparoscopy, and a miscarriage, and thanks to Clomid, a fertility medication. My pregnancies went well, but both girls, each at 8.5 pounds, were delivered by C-section. The births were positive experiences. My older daughter was able to rock her new sister in a rocking chair in the recovery room as my husband, parents, and brother celebrated. I did have the "blues," yet they passed each time as my incision healed. All in all, my pregnancies, births, and postpartum experiences were positive. This only added to my outrage when I learned about perinatal mood and anxiety disorders. Everyone should have the right to an emotionally and physically healthy pregnancy and postpartum experience! And all healthcare providers should be screening and treating mental health illnesses the same way they do gestational diabetes or any other perinatal health concern.

My history of political activism served me well. I joined organizations and read books, attended conferences and trainings. Jane Honikman of Postpartum Support International told me about a woman in the East Bay, Shoshana Bennett, who was doing postpartum work. I called and asked if she would meet with me to make sure I was on the right track. Since that time, I have been a coordinator for Postpartum Support International, and served as the chair of PSI's Education and Training Committee. Creating curriculum, lecturing and providing trainings all over the United States, I have been honored to give keynote talks in Beijing and Shanghai, China; Jakarta, Indonesia; and Mexico City. I have worked as a consultant for both federal and local governmental perinatal programs. As part of PSI's educational committee, I am delighted to have been involved in the creation of our first educational video, *Healthy Mom, Happy Family* (see the Resources section). Most recently, I became nationally certified as a Perinatal Mental Health Provider. Currently I serve as a subject expert for the Certification Committee and also serve on the PSI Advisory Council.

This work has become my passion. I have never experienced so much personal and professional meaning and reward. I hope you will join us on this mission.

Two

Perinatal Psychiatric Illness

Some of the words or terms we use are medically based. We have included an Appendix in the back of the book to clarify and explain the meanings of these words.

Perinatal mood and anxiety disorders (PMADs) occur during pregnancy and the first year after birth. The terms *prenatal* or *antenatal* (during pregnancy) and *postpartum* or *postnatal* (after birth) are also used to describe more specifically when these conditions occur. These mood and anxiety disorders are triggered mainly by hormonal changes, which then affect brain chemicals called neurotransmitters. Genetics, as well as life stressors, such as moving, illness, poor partner support, financial problems, and social isolation, are certainly also important and can negatively affect a person's mental state. Parents who have had perinatal losses and fertility struggles are at an increased risk of experiencing a mental health challenge, as are parents who have adopted. LGBTQ (lesbian, gay, bisexual, transgender, questioning) parents are also at a higher risk of developing a PMAD due to discrimination and less social support. Military families also have an increased risk of postpartum depression. Understanding and attending to your risk factors can reduce a crisis. Strong emotional, social, and physical support will help recovery.

PMADs occur wherever babies are born. In a study in 2020 (Prom) it was found that perinatal depression in low- to middle-income countries was 25% compared to 7%–15% in high-income countries. Prenatal anxiety in low- to middle-income countries was 18% compared to 13% in high-income countries. Rates increased up to 34% during the COVID-19 pandemic (Chen, 2022).

Perinatal mood and anxiety disorders behave quite differently from other mood or anxiety disorders experienced at other times, because the hormones are going up and down. A woman with a PMAD often feels as if she's losing control, since she can never predict how she will feel at any given moment. For instance, at 8:00 a.m. she may be gripped with anxiety, at 10:00 a.m. feel almost normal, and at 10:30 a.m. become depressed.

Our clients who have had personal histories of depression tell us that perinatal depression feels very different from (and usually much worse than) depressions at other times in their lives. One of Shoshana's postpartum clients is a survivor of breast cancer. At a support group, she beautifully explained:

> *When I had cancer, I thought that was the worst experience I could ever have. I was wrong—this is. With cancer, I allowed myself to ask for and receive help, and expected to be depressed. My friends and family rallied around me, bringing me meals, cleaning my house, and giving me lots of emotional support. Now, during postpartum depression, I feel guilty asking for help and ashamed of my depression. Everyone expects me to feel happy and doesn't accept that this illness is just as real as cancer.*

Parents who experience these symptoms need to speak up and be persistent in getting proper care. In the past, these illnesses have been downplayed and even dismissed. Research has shown how important it is to treat perinatal mood and anxiety disorders for the health and well-being of the one suffering, baby, and entire family.

In 2017, the American College of Obstetricians and Gynecologists (ACOG) noted the seriousness of these illnesses.

"Perinatal mood and anxiety disorders are among the most common mental health conditions encountered by women of reproductive age. When left untreated, perinatal mood and anxiety disorders can have profound adverse effects on women and their children, ranging from increased risk of poor adherence to medical care, worsening of medical conditions, loss of interpersonal and financial resources, smoking and substance use, suicide, and infanticide" (Kendig, 2017).

Death by suicide is a leading cause of about 20% of postpartum deaths. Although maternal death rates from infection and bleeding have gone down, the rate of maternal deaths by suicide have remained high. Good treatment is essential (Chin, 2022).

Researchers are beginning to look at early risk factors to improve detection and guide treatment. An exciting study published in 2023 (Guintivano) examined genetic samples from all over the world. They found that major depression and postpartum depression may have specific genetic markers. A small study in China (Sheng, 2023) of women who had C-sections found that biomarkers in spinal fluid may predict PPD. We are hopeful these efforts will reduce suffering in the future.

Perinatal Mood and Anxiety Disorders

There are six principal perinatal mood and anxiety disorders, which are:

- Depression
- Bipolar disorder I or II (sometimes referred to as Bipolar Spectrum Disorder)
- Psychosis
- Obsessive-compulsive disorder (OCD)
- Panic disorder
- Post-traumatic stress disorder (PTSD)

This chapter explains each of these disorders, some of the most common symptoms, and risk factors. It is important to note that symptoms and their severity can change over the course of an illness. Also, when "personal or family history" is listed as a high risk factor, be aware that often relatives with these conditions may not have been formally diagnosed or treated.

The Psychiatric Issues of Pregnancy

Contrary to popular mythology, pregnancy is not always a happy, glowing experience. Pregnancy can lead to depression, bipolar disorder, anxiety and panic, post-traumatic stress disorder, obsessive-compulsive disorder, and even psychosis. This may be a reoccurrence of a previous illness, or a new onset of illness. Approximately 15% to 23% of pregnant women experience depression (Wisner, 2013). These rates are even higher in teenagers and those living in poverty.

In a study of 10,000 new mothers in the United States, it was found that by the end of the first postpartum year, 1 in 5 women had developed postpartum depression. Of those women, 26.5% had histories of depression before pregnancy, 33.4% had their first occurrence of depression during pregnancy, and 40.1% developed postpartum depression as their first depression (Wisner, 2013).

It can be confusing that many of the normal symptoms of pregnancy are very similar to symptoms of depression. It is easy to ignore or dismiss these symptoms as just a normal part of pregnancy. It is important that symptoms be evaluated and treated, if they are outside the normal range. The following section provides some guidelines to determine if symptoms are caused by pregnancy or depression.

PREGNANCY	DEPRESSION
Mood up and down, teary	Mood mostly down, gloomy, hopeless
Self-esteem unchanged	Low self-esteem, guilt
Can fall asleep, physical problems disrupt sleep (bladder, heartburn), can fall back to sleep	May have trouble falling asleep, may have early morning wakening and difficulty falling back to sleep
Tires easily, rest refreshes and energizes	Rest does not help reduce fatigue
Feels pleasure, joy, and anticipation	Lack of joy or pleasure
Appetite increases	Appetite may decrease

Depression and Anxiety in Pregnancy

When symptoms of a mood or anxiety disorder make it difficult to function on a day-to-day basis, treatment is necessary. This may include traditional (counseling and medication), nontraditional methods (such as yoga or acupuncture), or any combination. What's important is to use whatever works best, so you feel like yourself again. Depression during pregnancy has been associated with less prenatal care, low birth weight (under 5.8 pounds) and preterm delivery (fewer than 37 weeks). Severe anxiety during pregnancy may cause harm to a growing fetus. This is partly because cortisol, a hormone released during stress, can cause constriction of the blood vessels in the placenta. Substance abuse is also common when PMADs go untreated during pregnancy, which is unhealthy for all concerned.

Some women become pregnant while taking medications for depression, anxiety, or other mental health problem. Many of these medications are considered acceptable during pregnancy, and recommended, if necessary, to keep the woman well (Janecka, 2018; Andrade, 2018; Momen, 2022).

Seek out a healthcare practitioner who is familiar with the current research about the safety of taking medications during pregnancy. Do not assume all healthcare providers are informed or up-to-date about treating mood or anxiety problems during pregnancy (refer to "Finding a Therapist or Medical Practitioner" in Chapter 3).

The likelihood of becoming ill again with a major depressive disorder (MDD) in women who discontinue their medication before pregnancy is between 50% and 75% (Cohen, 2006). In other words, only 25% to 50% of women who stopped taking medication before trying to get pregnant stayed well. The rate of relapse for MDD in those who discontinue medications at conception or in early pregnancy is 75%, with up to 60% relapsing in the first trimester. This means that most of the women who stopped medication once they discovered they were pregnant became ill again early in the pregnancy. In one study, 42% of women who discontinued medications at conception resumed medications at some time during their pregnancy (Cohen, 2004). In a more recent study it was noted that relapse was more likely in women who had a history of recurrent depression or severe depression. Counseling before a pregnancy and monitoring throughout pregnancy are recommended (Bayrampour, 2020).

Resources listed at the end of this book provide helpful guidelines regarding the use of medications.

Symptoms of Depression and Anxiety

- Sad mood
- Difficulty coping
- Irritability
- Lack of joy or pleasure, not looking forward to the future
- Guilt

- Excessive worry or fear
- Social withdrawal
- Appetite and sleep disturbances
- Exhaustion

Risk Factors

- Personal or family history of mental health problems (diagnosed or not)
- Lack of support
- Stopping psychiatric medication
- History of abuse, domestic violence
- Poverty
- Addiction
- Pregnancy with multiples
- History of pregnancy loss
- Thyroid problems

Stacey's Story

I had always wanted to be a mom. I was the oldest of four and took care of my brothers and sisters. We were all verbally abused, and I was treated for depression in high school and in my twenties. When I got pregnant, I immediately stopped my medication. It was a terrible pregnancy, and I became very depressed. I didn't eat well, I didn't feel like shopping for baby things, I didn't feel any of the joy and excitement I thought I would feel. I felt like I wouldn't be able to be a good mom and that I'd made a big mistake.

Finally, after being diagnosed with postpartum depression, I went back on medication. I began to feel better, shop for the baby, and most importantly enjoy her. When I wanted to get pregnant again, I consulted a psychiatrist trained in issues related to medications in pregnancy. Together we discussed the risks of being on medication compared to the risks to me, the baby, and my toddler if I went off medication and became depressed again. I decided to stay on the medication during the pregnancy. It was very different the second time. I really bonded with the baby growing inside me, and could enjoy him (and his sister) after he was born. I really wish I could've enjoyed the first pregnancy.

After the Birth, "Baby Blues"—Not a Disorder

The term *Baby Blues* is used to describe *mild* mood swings that occur during the first two weeks after birth. This is not considered a disorder since the majority of mothers experience it.

Baby Blues

- Occurs in about 80% of mothers
- Always begins during first week postpartum
- Should be gone by three weeks postpartum

Symptoms

- Moodiness
- Crying
- Sadness
- Worry
- Lack of concentration
- Forgetfulness
- Feelings of dependency

Causes

- Rapid hormonal changes
- Physical and emotional stress of birthing
- Physical discomforts
- Emotional letdown after pregnancy and birth
- Awareness and fear about increased responsibility
- Fatigue and sleep deprivation

- Disappointments including the birth, partner support, nursing, and the baby

Deborah's Story

For about a week and a half after my baby was born I would cry for no reason at all. Sometimes I would feel overwhelmed, especially when I was up at night with my son. Once I even thought that I had made a big mistake having a child. I felt resentment toward my husband since his life stayed pretty much the same and mine was turned upside down. When I started going to the mother's club at two weeks, I felt so relieved that all these other moms felt the same way.

Deborah's Treatment

Since Deborah was experiencing normal postpartum adjustment, she did not require any formal treatment. All she needed in order to enjoy her new life was a combination of socializing with other moms, more sleep, taking time to care for herself, and working out a plan of sharing child and household responsibilities with her husband.

Depression and Anxiety Postpartum

This section describes depression and anxiety that occur in the first year after birth. The onset of illness is usually gradual, but it can be rapid and begin any time during that first year. For parents who adopt, that first year begins when the baby enters the home. The adoption process itself is often stressful and anxiety-producing even before the baby joins the family.

Symptoms May Include

- Excessive worry or fear
- Irritability or short temper
- Feeling overwhelmed and unable to cope
- Difficulty making decisions

- Sadness
- Hopelessness
- Feelings of guilt
- Sleep problems (difficulty falling or staying asleep, or sleeping too much)
- Fatigue or exhaustion
- Physical symptoms or complaints without apparent physical cause
- Discomfort around the baby or a lack of feeling toward the baby
- Loss of focus and concentration (may miss appointments, for example)
- Loss of interest or pleasure, lower sex drive
- Changes in appetite, significant weight loss or gain

Risk Factors

- From 50% to 80% risk if previous postpartum depression/anxiety
- Depression or anxiety during pregnancy
- Personal or family history of depression, anxiety, and/or obsessive-compulsive disorder
- Abrupt weaning
- Perinatal loss (miscarriage, abortion, stillbirth, SIDS, or other loss of baby)
- Social isolation or poor support
- History of premenstrual syndrome (PMS) or premenstrual dysphoric disorder (PMDD)
- Negative mood changes while taking birth control pills or fertility medication
- Thyroid dysfunction
- Stopping psychiatric medication

Lori's Story

I was so excited about having our baby girl. My pregnancy had gone smoothly. I had been warned about the "Blues," but I just couldn't shake the tears and sadness that seemed to get deeper and darker every day. My appetite was nonexistent. Although I forced myself to eat because I was nursing. I lost about thirty pounds the first month. At night I was having trouble sleeping. My husband and baby would be asleep but I would have one worry after another going through my head. I was exhausted. I felt like my brain had been kidnapped. I couldn't make decisions, couldn't focus, and didn't want to be left alone with the baby.

I wanted to run away. I withdrew from friends and felt guilty about not returning phone calls, emails, or texts. I couldn't understand why I felt so bad; I had the greatest, most supportive husband, a home I loved, and the beautiful baby I had always wanted. At times I felt close to her, but at other times I felt like I was just going through the motions—she could have been someone else's child. I thought I was the worst mother and wife on the face of the earth.

Lori's Treatment

Lori began psychotherapy, a sleep medication prescribed by a psychiatrist, and transcranial magnetic stimulation (TMS) for depression. After four weeks of daily TMS sessions, the depression lifted. She began taking regular breaks to take care of herself, nibbled every few hours until her appetite returned, and also began taking a pharmaceutical-grade omega-3 supplement. She started attending a postpartum depression support group and met other moms with similar stories. After a few months she felt like herself.

Obsessive-Compulsive Disorder (OCD)

Risk of new onset of OCD and worsening of OCD increase during the perinatal period. Rates for a new onset of OCD in pregnancy vary from 2% to 22%. There is a slightly higher risk of new onset as well as worsening postpartum, where rates have been reported to up to 24%. Of those, over 38% also suffer from depression. Pregnancies impacted by OCD are at higher risk for poor obstetrical and neonatal outcomes including high blood pressure, preeclampsia, poor growth of the fetus and preterm birth (Hudepohl, 2022).

Symptoms May Include

- Intrusive, repetitive, and persistent thoughts or mental pictures
- Thoughts and/or images, often about the baby being hurt or killed
- Tremendous sense of horror and disgust about these thoughts/images
- Thoughts, possibly accompanied by behaviors to reduce the anxiety (for example, hiding knives or avoiding high places)
- Counting (diapers), checking (the baby's breathing, windows, door locks), cleaning or other repetitive behaviors
- Fear of germs
- Excessive fears about her own or baby's health

Risk Factor

Personal or family history of obsessive-compulsive disorder (diagnosed or not)

Tanya's Story

Each time I went near the balcony I would clutch my baby tightly until I was in a room with the door closed. Only then did

I know he was safe one more time from me dropping him over the edge. The bloody scenes I would envision horrified me. Passing the steak knives in the kitchen triggered images of my stabbing the baby, so I asked my husband to hide the knives. I never bathed my baby alone since I was afraid I might drown him.

Although I didn't think I would ever really hurt my baby son, I never trusted myself alone with him. I was terrified I would "snap" and actually carry out one of these scary thoughts. If my baby got sick, it would be all my fault, so I would clean and clean to make sure there were no germs. Although I had always been more careful than other people, now I would check the locks on the windows and doors many times a day.

Tanya's Treatment

Tanya found that the most recommended psychotherapy for OCD is cognitive behavioral therapy with exposure and response prevention (CBT with ERP). It is considered safe and very effective in pregnancy and postpartum.

After meeting with Tanya twice individually, her therapist suggested that her husband join her in the next session. Tanya needed reassurance that her husband knew she wasn't "crazy" and that she would never really harm the baby. It wasn't important to tell him the specific graphic thoughts, so she referred to them generally as "scary thoughts." After being educated, her husband's aggravation with her being "nervous all the time" subsided.

Tanya started taking an antidepressant, and soon the scary thoughts were occurring less frequently. She began taking a pharmaceutical-grade omega-3 supplement and nibbled or drank nutritious food every few hours until her appetite returned. Her therapist suggested that she wait another few weeks to join a support group, until she felt less vulnerable about hearing the anxieties of others. In the meantime, she was given the names and numbers of a few women to connect with who had recovered from postpartum OCD.

Panic Disorder

Anxiety disorders occur in about 15.8% of pregnant women and 17% of newly postpartum women (Fairbrother, 2016).

Symptoms May Include

- Episodes of extreme anxiety
- Shortness of breath, chest pain, sensations of choking or smothering, dizziness
- Hot or cold flashes, trembling, rapid heartbeat, numbness or tingling sensations
- Restlessness, agitation, or irritability
- Fear of going crazy, dying, or losing control
- Panic attack may awaken from sleep
- Often no identifiable trigger for the panic
- Excessive worry or fears (including fear of more panic attacks)

Risk Factors

- Personal or family history of anxiety or panic disorder (diagnosed or not)
- Thyroid dysfunction

Chris's Story

At about three weeks postpartum I stopped leaving my house at all except for pediatrician appointments. I was afraid I might have a panic attack in the store and not be able to take care of my baby. I never knew when that wave would begin washing over me and I would "lose it." The windows had to be open all the time or else I thought I would suffocate if I had an attack.

The first time I had a panic attack I thought I was having a major heart attack. A friend drove me to the emergency room and the doctor on call told me it was only stress. He gave me some medicine but I was too afraid to take it. I went home feeling stupid, like I had made a big deal out of nothing.

Everyone told me that breastfeeding would relax me, but it did just the opposite. I never knew how much milk my baby was getting and that really worried me. Sometimes when my milk would let down I would get a panic attack. The first therapist I saw told me I must have had issues bonding with my own mother, but I knew that wasn't true, and I didn't see that therapist again. On many nights I woke up in a sweat, with my heart beating so fast and hard. My head was racing with anxious thoughts about who would take care of the baby when I died. I thought I was going crazy. I was so scared.

Chris's Treatment

Chris had her first therapy appointment over the telephone since she felt she could not go outside. Driving was too scary for her, especially in tunnels and over bridges. Her husband drove her to her next session, following a route that avoided those obstacles. Chris needed to sit near the door during the appointment just in case she felt the need to run outside for some air. She began stress management classes and her medical provider ordered lab work to rule out medical causes of her panic. Her therapist urged her to sleep for at least half the night, every night. Chris's husband began taking care of the baby for the first half of the night on a regular basis. Chris noticed immediately how sleep lowered her stress level. She attended an infant massage class, which also helped.

Psychosis

Psychosis is a serious illness in which a person loses touch with reality. It occurs in 2.6 per thousand perinatal women (Michalczyk, 2023).

Onset is usually within the first two weeks after the woman gives birth. With postpartum psychotic disorder there is a 5% suicide and 4% infanticide rate (Brockington, 2017).

Symptoms May Include

- Seeing, hearing, or feeling things that others do not (for example, hearing the voice of God, or the devil, or getting "secret messages" from the television)
- Delusional thinking (for example, about the infant's death, denial of birth, or the need to kill the baby)
- Mania
- Saying things that don't make sense to others
- Confusion
- Rage
- Paranoia
- Symptoms that come and go (such as, she may seem normal one minute, and hearing voices the next minute)

Risk Factors

- Personal or family history of psychosis or bipolar disorder—40%–50% increased risk
- Schizophrenia (diagnosed or not)
- Previous postpartum psychotic or bipolar episode
- Hormone shifts, obstetrical complications, sleep deprivation, and increased environmental stress

Mike's Story

My wife Gloria had a great pregnancy and a long labor. We were thrilled to have our first child, a son. But within days of his birth my wife began to withdraw into her own world. She became less and less communicative and she became more and more confused and suspicious. I almost had to carry her into the therapist's office; by that time she could hardly speak or answer questions, nor write her name on the forms her therapist gave us. I was told to take her to the hospital immediately.

When we arrived at the hospital, she became fearful and then violent. She ended up in restraints. Fortunately, she responded pretty quickly to the antipsychotic medication, and was able to come home after about a week. She continued to improve.

Over time and under the doctor's guidance, Gloria was able to wean herself off her medication.

We had always wanted two kids, so we consulted with our therapist and psychiatrist. With careful planning, we now have our second child and a very different story to tell.

Gloria's Treatment
After being released from the hospital, Gloria continued therapy and saw the psychiatrist, who carefully monitored her medication. Gloria worked to understand and process what had happened to her. Eventually she joined an online postpartum support group specifically for survivors of postpartum psychosis, which was quite helpful. The group leader also gave her the names and numbers of women near where she lives who had "been there" and who wanted to offer support in person.

Post-traumatic Stress Disorder (PTSD)

PTSD can occur following life-threatening or injury-producing events such as sexual abuse or assault, or traumatic childbirth. It occurs in up to 6% of women. Rates are higher (up to 30%) in parents who have a child in the intensive care unit. According to Beck (2018), 45% of mothers perceived their labor and delivery experiences as traumatic and up to 9% had sufficient symptoms to be given a diagnosis of PTSD. Witnessing a traumatic event can also trigger PTSD.

Symptoms May Include

- Recurrent nightmares
- Extreme anxiety
- Reliving past traumatic events (for example, sexual, physical, and emotional events, and childbirth)
- Avoidance of potential triggers (like returning to the hospital, or seeing her healthcare provider

Risk Factors

- Past traumatic events or witnessing trauma
- Traumatic birth
- Severe physical complication or injury related to pregnancy or childbirth
- Baby in the neonatal intensive care unit (NICU)

Jennifer's Story

During the delivery it all came flooding back. I felt terrorized and vulnerable. I thought I had already dealt with the abuse in my childhood. It seemed that all the years of therapy were a waste of time and money. I was so embarrassed for losing control during labor. I was angry that what happened to me as a kid was still affecting me after all this time.

My therapist told me the nightmares and flashbacks would go away, but I just didn't know. It was so real—like the abuse was happening again over and over. I couldn't even leave my poor husband alone with my baby. I got the sick feeling that I couldn't trust even him. I was so messed up. I thought maybe I'd never be a normal mother.

Jennifer's Treatment

Jennifer hired a postpartum doula who took care of her and the baby for two months. Having this trusted female companion with her almost everywhere she went gave Jennifer comfort. She began weekly therapy sessions and eventually joined a support group. She and her therapist agreed that she did not need medication at this point.

Bipolar Disorder I or II (sometimes referred to as Bipolar Spectrum Disorder)

Also known as manic depression, bipolar disorders are characterized by moodswings from very high (mania), or high (hypomania) to low mood (depression). Treatment occurs more frequently during an episode of depression and is commonly misdiagnosed as a depressive disorder, rather than a bipolar disorder.

Symptoms

- Mania (bipolar I) or hypomania (low level of mania in bipolar II; see the Appendix for a description)
- Depression (almost always present)
- Rapid and severe mood swings

Risk Factor

Personal or family history of bipolar disorder (diagnosed or not)

Tammy's Story

After my son was born I was happier than I'd ever been in my life. Everything felt wonderful. Everyone told me I should sleep when my baby slept, but I was too excited to sleep. I was really proud of myself that I kept the house spotless, took care of my baby, and was still able to look great. My husband was pleased that dinner would always be ready for him when he came home. I was handling everything like a supermom, and felt on top of the world. After about two weeks my world started spinning out of control. I crashed. I started crying very easily and then a minute later I hated my husband and wanted a divorce. I started doing weird things like tape recording the baby all day so I could study his cries. I would also record my thoughts since I believed they were profound and should be documented. My head would not slow down for a second. It was exhausting.

Tammy's Treatment

Unfortunately, Tammy was first misdiagnosed as having postpartum depression, and she was given an antidepressant. She became more manic. She finally found a psychiatrist who diagnosed her as having postpartum bipolar disorder. Tammy was prescribed an antipsychotic medication for a few weeks to sedate her enough to sleep at night when her husband was watching the baby. She was also put on a mood stabilizer. To help reset her "internal clock," she started wearing special lenses (see Resources section) each night before she went to bed, and soon was able to decrease the medication. In therapy, she began to understand what had happened to her, and she set up realistic expectations for herself as a mother and wife. She started taking a pharmaceutical-grade omega-3 supplement and made sure to eat regularly even when she wasn't hungry. Eventually her moods became stable. When she and her husband are ready to have another baby, they will create a treatment plan with her psychiatrist for pregnancy and postpartum.

Consequences of *Untreated* Depression in Parents

The American Academy of Pediatrics states that untreated illness "leads to increased costs of medical care, inappropriate medical treatment of the infant, discontinuation of breastfeeding, family dysfunction, and an increased risk of abuse and neglect. Postpartum depression, specifically, adversely affects this critical early period of infant brain development. Perinatal depression is an example of an adverse childhood experience that has potential long-term adverse health complications for the mother, her partner, the infant, and the mother-infant dyad" (Earls, 2019).

Suicide is a leading cause of maternal deaths. It occurs all over the world and accounts for approximately 20% of postpartum deaths in the U.S. (Kendig, 2017; CDC 2022). In a large study in 2024 (Yu) it was found that suicide risk was highest in women with depression in the perinatal period, up to one year postpartum.

There is a tremendous amount of data that shows what a negative impact untreated parental depression has on fetuses, babies, and other children in the home. That impact may continue through childhood and into the teen years.

Fifty percent of children of depressed moms will have depression by the end of adolescence. Children of depressed parents are more likely to suffer from childhood psychiatric disturbance, behavior problems, poor social functioning, and impaired cognitive and language development. When a depressed parent goes untreated, every member of the family and all the relationships within the family are affected. The quicker the parent is treated, the better it is for the entire family. The longer the depression remains, the more likely the children and family are to suffer depression. In the Netsi 2018 study, some women with persistent depression continued to have significant symptoms up to 11 years after childbirth.

These are very sobering statistics; however, we want to emphasize the heading of this section. It's *untreated* parental depression that causes problems. The takeaway message is, of course, get treated right away to help ensure a healthy family.

Remember that the goal of treatment is not just to feel *better*, but to feel *well*.

Perinatal Loss

No matter how a pregnancy ends (miscarriage, abortion, stillbirth, sudden infant death syndrome), whether by nature or by choice, depression and anxiety may follow due to physiological factors as well as emotional. Grief should be addressed through counseling, and other types of treatment may also be useful. Although miscarriage occurs frequently (over 20% of pregnancies), often it's not discussed. Many people are uncomfortable talking about death and loss, so it's important to find support and know you are not alone. Those who have experienced any neonatal loss need to be monitored carefully for distress in future pregnancies and the postpartum period.

When there is a pregnancy loss, both parents may suffer. Each person grieves differently, and counseling for the couple can often be helpful. Moms go through an immediate physiological and emotional reaction. Partners often feel they need to be "strong," and the "rock," and they are often the ones taking care of details and are on "autopilot." This stoic response is sometimes perceived as a lack of caring or grieving. This can cause hurt and tension in the relationship.

In a study from the United Kingdom, 36% of dads suffered from severe anxiety at six weeks after a pregnancy loss. Interestingly, dads were found to have more depression than the moms at thirteen months after the loss. It may be that as the mom's depression post-loss improves, the partner falls apart. Couples really need good communication to work as a team and support each other. Among other measures, the support plan should include nutrition, sleep, social support, possible medication, or alternative treatments.

Three

Perinatal Disorders

If you are suffering, this chapter is for you. In the chapters to follow, we will discuss the role of practitioners, partners, and other family members in helping with recovery.

Among those we treat are workers in the healthcare and educational professions, such as MDs, nurses, daycare and preschool providers, teachers, and therapists, to name a few. We often hear from them, "This can't be happening to me! I take care of everyone else in crisis." What we tell them is that our brain doesn't care what we do for a living! No one is immune. No matter what the educational or socioeconomic level, culture, religion, or personality, wherever babies are being born, the statistics remain consistent.

Those who suffer perinatal emotional difficulty experience their emotional pain in many different ways. Here are some of the common feelings they express:

No one has ever felt as bad as I do.
I'm all alone. No one understands.
I'm a failure as a woman, mother, and wife.
I'll never be myself again.
I've made a terrible mistake.
I'm on an emotional roller coaster.
I'm losing it.
I wasn't cut out to be a parent.
I can't cope.

Please know that every parent may experience these feelings at varying levels. Some may feel all of them, and others may feel only a few. You might also recognize some of your symptoms listed in Chapter 2.

Finding a Therapist or Medical Practitioner

We encourage you to contact Postpartum Support International (PSI) at 800-944-4PPD (800-944-4773) or postpartum.net to locate a therapist who has training in the field of perinatal mental health. PSI, along with other organizations, provides specialized training in perinatal mood and anxiety disorders. We have not found any graduate training that fully covers this material. Do not assume (as many insurance companies would like you to believe) that someone who has expertise in working with depression or anxiety is knowledgeable about the unique aspects of perinatal mood and anxiety disorders.

Most insurance companies have coverage for mental health. It is usually less expensive if you see a provider on their "panel." Sometimes an insurance company is willing to add a specialist to its provider list or pay for you to see one. If your insurance company will pay only if you see providers on their list, here are screening questions to help you determine their knowledge in this area. It's important to ask these questions, even if the therapist considers himself or herself knowledgeable. If you don't have the energy to deal with the insurance company or to screen professionals, ask a support person to do this for you. Medical practitioners should be asked if they are comfortable with psychiatric medication (if needed) during pregnancy and breastfeeding.

- *What training have you received specifically in perinatal mood and anxiety disorders?* A therapist who specializes in PMADs should have had a minimum of two full days of training on this particular topic.

- *Do you belong to any organization dedicated to education about perinatal mood and anxiety disorders?* Someone committed to working in this field should belong to at least one of these organizations: Postpartum Support International, Marcé Society, North American Society for Psychosocial OB/GYN.
- *What books do you recommend to women with prenatal or postpartum depression or anxiety?* Someone with expertise should be able to name several books specifically about understanding and treating perinatal mood and anxiety disorders.
- *What is your theoretical orientation?* Research has shown the most effective types of therapy for your condition are cognitive-behavioral (CBT) and interpersonal psychotherapy (IPT). During the COVID-19 pandemic a Canadian study (Van Lieshout, 2021) of postpartum women found that a one-day CBT online workshop improved mood, bonding, and social support. If you are experiencing a life crisis; long-term intensive psychoanalysis is not appropriate.

If you are unable to find a therapist with expertise, interview until you find someone who is compassionate and willing to learn. If you do not think a practitioner is helping you, move on! Be a good consumer. Shop around until you feel satisfied that you are in capable hands.

The Truth of the Matter

As you face the challenge of a postpartum mood or anxiety disorder, remind yourself of these truths:

- *I will recover!*
  We have never met a parent who, after proper treatment, did not recover.
- *I am not alone!*

One in five women and one in ten dads will experience a PMAD.

- ***This is not my fault!***
  You did not create this; it is a real illness.
- ***I am a good parent!***
  Even if you are hospitalized, you are still making sure your baby is provided for. The fact that you are trying to improve the quality of your life and your family's proves you are a good parent.
- ***It is essential for me to take care of myself!***
  It is your job to take care of yourself so you can get better and take care of your family.
- ***I am doing the best I can.***
  No matter what your current level of functioning, you are taking steps, regardless of how small they seem. Good for you!

Depression may interfere with your ability to believe these truths, so it is important to say them frequently, as if you really mean them. As you recover, this exercise will become easier.

Basic Mom Care

Women today are expected to be supermoms and do it all. There is a lot of pressure to have a perfect baby who never cries, a clean and well-organized home, and a happy, supportive partner. Even when there are helpful people around, it's common to feel uncomfortable asking for help. We often hear the expression, "It takes a village," but many feel that asking for or needing help is a sign of weakness. You deserve to be well no matter how much help it takes.

Finding Support People

Very often when we are in crisis, we overlook the people around us who can be of help and support. People can support you in different ways, and all types of support are needed. Physical support can be help with cooking, cleaning, caring for the baby, shopping, or taking you for a walk or to an appointment. Emotional support may include sitting and listening, hugging, and giving encouraging words. Accept all the help that's offered and ask for more.

This is a brainstorming exercise. Write down everyone who comes to mind, regardless of the type of support he or she may be able to give you. If possible, do this exercise with a support person. Keep this list of supporters' names and phone numbers handy. Do not assume that because someone is in a helping profession or is family, he or she will be helpful or understanding. Find and surround yourself with nonjudgmental, caring support.

Here are some places where our clients have found support. Think about how these sources might help you the best:

- Partner
- Friends
- Family and extended family
- Neighbors
- Coworkers
- Religious/faith/spiritual/cultural communities
- Professionals (including doulas, lactation consultants, nannies, housekeepers, home visitors)
- 24-hour hotlines, such as the National Maternal Mental Health Hotline—24/7, free, confidential support before, during, and after pregnancy. Call or text 833-TLC-MAMA (833-852-6262.) TTY users can use a preferred relay service or dial 711 and then 833-852-6262.
- Helplines such as Postpartum Support International's warmline. Leave a message or text 800-944-4773, #1 for

English or #2 for Spanish and get a call back (see Resources section).

- Online postpartum depression message boards (see Resources section)
- PMAD support groups (such as postpartum.net)

Eating

Often those with perinatal depression and anxiety crave sweets and carbohydrates. If you can eat something nutritious, especially protein, each time you feed the baby, you can help keep your blood sugar level even. This will contribute to keeping your mood stable. We understand this may be difficult if you are experiencing a lack of appetite, so do the best you can. If you have trouble eating, try drinking your food—for example, protein shakes or drinks. Avoid caffeine.

Ask a support person or delivery service to shop for things like yogurt, sliced deli meat and cheese, hardboiled eggs, precut vegetables, fruit, and nuts. Better yet, if they are not already offering, ask people to bring you food. Don't forget to drink water—dehydration can increase anxiety. Appetite problems are quite common with perinatal depression and anxiety. Please tell your health practitioner about any major appetite or weight changes. It might be helpful to consult a nutritionist who is familiar with depression and anxiety when you have the energy.

A study of over 1,000 women looked at the effect of diet on depression and anxiety (Bodnar, 2005). Women (across age, socioeconomic status, education, and health habits) who ate a diet high in vegetables, fruit, meat, fish, and whole grains had less depression and anxiety. Women who ate a diet of processed or fried foods, refined grains, sugary products, and beer had higher rates of depression and anxiety.

Sleeping

Mood is severely affected by poor sleep or lack of sleep. Sleep-deprived parents are more depressed, irritable, and anxious and are significantly at risk for PMADs. Nighttime sleep is the most valuable sleep in helping you recover. Sleep is necessary to restore brain health. Ideally, the brain needs at least 7 hours of uninterrupted sleep each night. You need to be "off duty" physically, emotionally, and psychologically for at least a few hours each night. Make a plan with a support person for how and when you will get your turn for sleep. You may need earplugs, a fan, or something to mask baby noises. However you choose to make it work for you, quality sleep is essential for mental health.

Beware of speakers and authors (even those with big names) who denounce any sleep plan except for baby right next to mother, nursing all night, every night. Since we are ethical professionals, we will not mention names, but you will recognize them. If you look closely, often these speakers and authors are paid by specific parenting organizations to push their agendas. The data they present is heavily skewed to support the paying organizations' message, without any regard to mother's mental health. Do not trust any professional, even one who offers data, who says there is only one right way, or a "best" way to sleep (or feed) and puts down any other way. We believe that whatever plans work for you and your family are the right ways, and one size never fits all. We are all individuals. Sometimes parents sleep better with their babies in co-sleepers, sometimes in the next room with a monitor, sometimes partial breastfeeding mixed with bottle feeding, sometimes with another person completely on duty. Find what works for you, and do that. And give yourself a pat on the back for trusting your intuition and creativity!

Remember, it is your job to take care of yourself. No one can do it for you. Even if you cannot arrange for this nightly, a few nights a week will help. If you are able to nap in the day, do so, but naps do not replace nighttime sleep. Sleep problems occur frequently with mood and anxiety disorders. Poor prenatal sleep has been associated with postpartum depression (Felder, 2023).

PMADs can cause sleep disturbances, and sleep disturbances interfere with recovery. Work on developing good sleep habits (also called sleep hygiene). LowBlueLights.com is the only company we have found that has studied the effectiveness of their lenses for promoting sleep, including for perinatal use. Consider getting a pair of these special glasses to wear for a couple of hours before bed. If possible, take a walk with your baby in the morning to get sunlight that will help restore your internal body clock. If you're not using these special lenses, turn off your computer and phone an hour before bed (these lights and stimulation can keep you awake). If you are unable to sleep at night when everyone else is sleeping, please talk to your health practitioner.

Physical Activity

Even a few minutes of brisk physical activity can help your mood. When you are physically able to be active, find something you are willing to do (for example, walking, dancing, or bike riding). If the thought of walking around the block is overwhelming, start slowly and work up. It will get easier as you feel better. If you know you would feel better if you did the activity, but it is hard to mobilize yourself, designate a support person or buddy to encourage you and participate with you. Pregnant and postpartum women who get some exercise (including walking with a stroller) cope better and have a reduction in depression.

If you have sleep problems or are very sleep deprived, do not do intense aerobics—this can actually make your sleep condition worse. Wait until you have had at least a couple of weeks of good sleep before you resume or begin a heavy exercise program.

Taking Breaks

The myth is that if we really love our children enough, we shouldn't need breaks from them or have fun without them. This certainly isn't the case! Many have bought into the idea that taking time for ourselves is selfish and bad, and therefore we feel guilty when we even think we need a break. (Dads are generally better at taking breaks than moms are.) There's no other job that's 24/7. The truth is that all good parents take breaks—that's how they stay good parents. We strongly recommend that you get regularly scheduled time off each week for a minimum of two hours at a time (pleasure only— this does not include chores and errands). For every job other than being a parent, breaks are mandated by law, and you'd expect much more time off.

If you don't recharge your batteries, you'll be running on empty. You are not the only one who can care for the baby. Partners and family members, for instance, should be given alone time to bond with the baby too. This experience is important for the baby, and it can be done more easily with you somewhere else. Everyone wins.

If you are not able to leave the house, go to another room and use earplugs or headphones. Or maybe your support person can leave the house with the baby and give you time alone.

Going Outside

When you are depressed or anxious, the four walls feel as if they're closing in. The world feels darker and smaller. You tend to fold in emotionally and physically (as in crossing your arms, hunching over, and fixing your gaze downward).

We encourage you to go outside your home, look up at the sky, stand up straight, put your arms at your sides, and breathe. You don't have to actually go anywhere. Just go outside once a day, even if this means standing outside your front door in your bathrobe.

Surround Yourself with Positive

Avoid reading or listening to the news, because it is often depressing or violent. If you want to watch a movie, choose a comedy. Avoid tragic or violent films. Open the curtains and let the sunlight in. If you are anxious, listen to soothing music. If you are depressed, try music with a good beat that gets your body moving. As much as possible, be around positive people who encourage, smile, and support.

Caring for the Baby

Depending on the level of depression, you may need someone to do most, if not all, of the baby care. A support person, such as a family member, doula, nanny, or friend, can be with you when your partner is not. Very gradually you can increase your participation with the baby care as your support person keeps you company.

Even though at first you may feel like a robot just going through the motions without joy, it is still good for you to experience yourself doing some "parent" tasks and interacting with the baby. Your feelings of competence and confidence will increase, and eventually you will be able to enjoy your day. Smile, touch, and interact with your baby as much as you're able. Once you're up to it, you might find it helpful to sign up for an infant massage or baby swim class. These types of classes promote bonding.

Scripts

You may not know what you need when a support person asks, "What can I do?" It's all right to say, "I don't know what I need right now. I just know I feel awful." However, don't assume anyone can read your mind. You are most likely to get what you need if you ask for it.

Try giving your partner, family, and friends a script to guide them in how to best support you. For example, when you are experiencing anxiety, it will not be helpful to hear, "Just calm down and relax." Instead, try giving them suggestions of what to say and do:

I am sorry you are suffering.

We will get through this.

I am here for you.

(Hug).

This will pass.

A script does not detract from the genuineness of caring and love. On the contrary, it will give your support people an effective way to give you what you need. People who love you want you to get better. They will be relieved to know what will help.

For Those with Anxiety, Fear, or Extreme Worry

Be sure to avoid caffeine and keep your blood sugar level even (see the section titled "Eating"). For many with anxiety or obsessions, information provides fuel for worry. Turn off the TV news, and don't read the news. Don't read books, magazines, or online information if you find it makes you more anxious. Avoid all media—including social media—if it fuels your worry, fear, or guilt. If you watch a movie, select a comedy. Find activities that can soothe or distract you, rather than those that stir up anxiety.

Preventing Too Much Stimulation

When the usual sights, sounds, and daily activity feel like too much, it is important to adjust your surroundings. Remember, you are in recovery. Treating yourself well can greatly boost your recovery. Don't push yourself. If, for instance, going to a family event seems overwhelming (even if you have had fun at this event in the past), you probably should not go, or your time there should at least be limited. Trust yourself. As you recover, you'll be able to handle more.

It's common to feel hypersensitive to stimulation of all kinds—visual (seeing), auditory (hearing), and kinesthetic (touch). If this is happening, it may be soothing to lower the light in your house. (If you are feeling more depressed than anxious, try brightening your house with more light—open your curtains and add lamps, for example.) As long as you can hear what you need to, try wearing earplugs or headphones during the day to muffle unnecessary noise. You may become more sensitive to touch—for instance, clothing may rub, scratch, or itch. Be compassionate with yourself and do what you need to in order to be comfortable.

Myths About Using Breast Milk

Myth: "I can't be a good mom unless I breastfeed my baby."

The truth is there is no one right way to feed your baby. Whatever works for you and your family is the right way. There is a tremendous amount of pressure on new moms in our society to breastfeed exclusively, regardless of physical or emotional obstacles. We believe that one size never fits all.

Whether you feed your baby breast milk (from breast or bottle) or formula, this has no relationship to how much you love your child or what kind of mother you are.

There are advantages and disadvantages to both breastfeeding and bottle feeding, and some combination of the two may work for you as well. For instance, having a support person bottle feed with formula or breast milk so you can be off duty is a responsible choice for your family's well-being. Don't allow yourself to be guilt-tripped!

Be prepared for intrusive and inappropriate questions and comments about how you're feeding your baby. This may happen anywhere—for example, out in public, at your health practitioner's office, in a moms' group, or at a family gathering. If any person, whether lay or professional, seems judgmental about the plan you've chosen, remind yourself that you have made the best decision you can for you and your family. You can ignore the question or comment or change the subject. Alternatively, you can say, "It's none of your business," "I can't breastfeed. I have a life-threatening illness," "I chose not to," or "My doctor told me I can't."

Women who breastfeed in public may also experience criticism. Be prepared to respond to comments like, "Why don't you do that in the bathroom?" One great response is, "I don't eat in the bathroom, and neither does my son."

Remember, you are entitled to respond any way you need to in order to get people off your back. You have nothing to apologize about, and you do not owe them an explanation. Good parents make sure their babies are fed. Period.

Here are some common myths we hear about parenting.

Myth: "My baby won't bond if I don't breastfeed."

If this were true, there would be whole generations of adults who never bonded with their mothers. Some women actually begin to bond with their babies when they stop breastfeeding. For women who are experiencing severe anxiety or pain related to breastfeeding, bottle feeding (formula or breast milk) or a combination of breastfeeding and bottle feeding may allow this time together to be more relaxed and enjoyable. Also, there are no rules about how to bottle feed. If you desire skin-to-skin contact, you can bottle feed bare-chested. Bottle feeding provides a chance for great eye contact and just as much bonding. Just because a mom is breastfeeding, she might not be using that as a bonding opportunity (being on her phone, for example). There are many chances throughout the day to bond with your baby, such as diaper changing, cuddling, bathing, smiling at your baby, and so on. Feeding is not the only time for bonding to take place. Bonding is an ongoing process of interaction. It goes far beyond how or what you feed your baby.

Myth: "My baby can sense my depression or anxiety."

Your baby cannot read your mind. Your thoughts or feelings will not damage your baby or the relationship with your baby. What babies can sense is temperature, hunger, wetness, and physical contact. Your baby will feel close to you regardless of depressed or anxious thoughts running through your head. It's your behavior that counts (smiling, talking, touching, and so on). Having a nondepressed caretaker in charge of the baby for part of the time will also help as you recover.

Myth: "Bonding happens only immediately at birth."

No adopted children would ever bond with their adoptive parents if this were true. There is no one magic moment of opportunity when bonding must happen, and no reason to worry about bonding if you were unable to touch or hold your baby immediately after delivery. Even if your depression or anxiety has made it difficult for you to care for your baby, it's never too late. Bonding is a process of familiarity, closeness, and comfort that continues for years.

Recovery

What will help each parent recover depends on the type, severity, and unique aspects of the illness and preferences for treatment. Whatever helps you get better quickly is what we recommend. In Chapter 7 we outline a few different treatment options that you may choose to do separately or in combination. Since medication is among the most common treatments for these disorders, we've discussed a few of the questions and concerns we hear most often.

Antidepressant Questions and Answers

Question: Will medication change my personality?

Answer: Depression and anxiety change your personality— people who are usually easygoing and stable may become irritable, moody, withdrawn, or worried. As the medication begins to work, you will begin to feel like yourself again. In a sense, medication restores you to your "normal" personality.

Question: How long will I have to take the medicine?

Answer: Treatment length varies, and is a decision between you and your prescribing practitioner. The general recommendation is to take a dose that gets you "back to yourself." Staying on the medication for the recommended time is critical to reduce your chances of having a relapse or recurrence of illness.

Question: Will I become dependent on the antidepressant?

Answer: Antidepressants are not addictive, but you should never stop taking them suddenly. Speak with your practitioner, who will guide the process of weaning yourself off the medication.

Question: What if I have side effects?

Answer: Many people experience no side effects at all. If side effects do occur, they are usually mild and temporary, lasting less than a week (nausea, fatigue, or shakiness, for instance). If you experience a decrease in sex drive or ability to orgasm, or if you feel more severe side effects or side effects that do not clear up after a week, contact your practitioner. Some need to try more than one antidepressant before they find the one that works best for them. To reduce the likelihood of side effects, it is helpful to start at a very low dose and slowly work up to the dosage that is effective for you.

Question: Which antidepressant is the right one for me?

Answer: In general, most people do well on most of the antidepressant medications. If you have previously been on a medication that was helpful, or if you have a blood relative doing well on a medication, that one would probably be the first choice. If you are anxious, a medication that may have a calming side effect might be chosen. If you have fatigue, a medication that may have an energizing side effect may be tried. The most important indicator is whether you begin to feel better over time.

Question: When will I feel better? How will I know if the medication is working?

Answer: Most of the newer antidepressants begin working within two weeks, while the older medications can take four to six weeks to work. It can take a number of weeks to gradually increase to the right dose. Here are some comments we have heard as the medicine begins working:

- *I'm not crying all the time.*
- *I have more patience and I'm not yelling as much.*
- *I'm singing in the shower again.*
- *My partner noticed I seem happier.*

- *I feel more motivated—I'm cooking for the family again.*
- *I'm enjoying the baby more.*
- *I'm not worrying as much—the little things aren't getting to me.*
- *I'm smiling and laughing more, and having fun.*
- *I'm answering email and phone calls again.*

Question: Won't medication be a crutch?

Answer: A crutch is a temporary tool that you use until you no longer need it. If you broke your foot you wouldn't think twice about using crutches to support you while your foot heals. Medication restores your brain chemistry to a normal state, allowing you to get back to feeling yourself and back to your life. As you become well, you and your provider will develop a plan to wean you off the medication. Additionally, medication can help you utilize psychotherapy more effectively.

Question: I want to breastfeed, but I don't want to take anything that will harm my baby. Can I take medication and breastfeed?

Answer: According to the professionals who have dedicated their careers to studying the safety of antidepressants while using breast milk, the answer is yes. When infant blood was examined, few, if any, metabolites of medication were found (di Scalea, 2009; Sprague, 2020). The use of medications to treat bipolar disorder (carbamezapine, lamotrigine, phenytoin, or valproate) have been found to have no adverse effects on infants. Babies exposed to medication through breast milk are as healthy and normal in all ways as babies not exposed to medication (Kronenfield, 2018). It's always important to remember that going untreated can affect the baby's health and is not a good option.

It's clear from the research that it is more important to receive proper treatment for mental health than whether the baby is fed with breast milk or formula. So if you think you will worry too much about your baby if you continue using breast milk while taking an antidepressant, it is better to wean yourself off the medication (slowly) rather than to go without treatment. Remember that the best gift you can give your baby is a happy, healthy mom. Often the fear about using breast milk while taking a medication goes away once the medication starts working, since the worry can be caused by the illness itself.

Question: I am pregnant and really depressed. Do I need to feel this way for the rest of my pregnancy?

Answer: Getting treatment is important for both you and the baby. Researchers have begun looking at the harmful effects of untreated depression and anxiety on the fetus. Also, if you are depressed or anxious in pregnancy, you may not be caring for yourself as you need to. This is not good for you or your developing baby. Many women self-medicate, for example with caffeine, tobacco (cigarettes or vaping), alcohol, drugs, or herbs, and this too can be harmful. Depression and/or anxiety can cause appetite changes that can make it difficult to maintain a healthy weight gain and good nutrition in pregnancy.

Counseling alone may be enough, but for some, medication is necessary to reduce serious symptoms. Antidepressants have been shown to be helpful for both depression and anxiety. No increased risk of miscarriage or malformations has been shown to result from taking these medications, even in the first trimester. Depression in pregnancy also puts you at high risk for postpartum depression, and can put the baby at risk for developmental delays. Being on medication through pregnancy and postpartum will significantly decrease this risk. According to the *American Journal of Obstetrics & Gynecology,*

"When a psychiatric condition necessitates pharmacotherapy (treatment with medication), the benefits of such therapy far outweigh the potential minimal risks" (Koren, 2012).

Question: I am embarrassed and ashamed about taking medication. Am I weak because I need a medication?

Answer: There is a stigma in many cultures about taking psychiatric medication. This stigma is based on ignorance and fear. Somehow it is presumed we can control our brain chemistry. If you had diabetes or a thyroid disorder you wouldn't expect (and no one would suggest) that you could will yourself to make more insulin or thyroid hormone. It's a strength to get help when we need it—not a weakness.

Taking medication is a personal choice. You are not required to share this information with others. Being private is not the same as being ashamed. However, once our clients begin to tell close family or friends, they are often surprised to find out how many of them are also on medication, or know someone who is. Whether or not you choose to take a medication, find people who will support your choices for wellness.

Four

Partners

This chapter is designed to provide support to you, the partner, regardless of your gender or marital status. For simplicity, we sometimes refer to the new mother as "wife." The sooner you become involved in the recovery process, and the greater your involvement, the more you both will benefit—together and separately. The more you understand what she is experiencing, the better supported she will feel. That will, in turn, speed recovery.

Having a baby brings changes to the whole family. Questions like, "Will I be a good parent?" and, "How can I best support my partner through this uncharted territory?" are normal and healthy to ask. This happens in all types of relationships—heterosexual, gay and lesbian couples, and adoptive parents. Having a baby changes things. Attention that had gone to the dad or partner now goes to the pregnancy. Fears, discomfort, and medical problems can affect intimacy. Once the baby is born, attention goes to the baby, and the couple relationship is on the back burner. We hear more these days about women's mood problems during pregnancy and postpartum, but we hear very little mentioned about the mental health of dads and partners. Dads and partners are important too!

Most often we are told the glowing side of parenthood— that you will feel instantly bonded and fall madly in love. That may happen, but often it's a process of getting to know this demanding stranger. There are losses associated with becoming a parent, and it's important to acknowledge and grieve them. It is normal for your relationship with your partner to change. If she's (or you've) been drooled on, spit up on, and sucked on all day, she (or you) may be "touched out." It's easy to feel rejected. Remind yourself it's not a personal rejection. You can no longer jump into bed, watch movies, or go out to dinner on a whim.

Some dads or partners may have a history of, or may be experiencing, a mood or anxiety disorder during the pregnancy. Depression and anxiety disorders (particularly obsessive-compulsive disorder) worsen during times of stress and sleep deprivation. It's important to assess your own risk going into a pregnancy. A large study that included research from many countries found that major risk factors for fathers were a history of mental illness, relationship dissatisfaction, wife's depression, financial instability, low education level, unemployment, and lack of social support (Ansari, 2021).

What do depressed or anxious dads look like? They look like dads. You can't tell by looking. When the mom is depressed, the rate of depression in her partner is significant—24% to 50%. A large multinational study (Rao, 2020) found that about 10% of dads experienced depression during the pregnancy. They found that overall in the first year postpartum 8.75% of fathers experienced depression, but depression increased to almost 10% between 3 and 6 months. Depressed fathers are nearly four times more likely to spank, and less than 50% of these dads report regularly reading to their 1-year-olds (Davis, 2011).

Evaluating multiple studies, prenatal anxiety in fathers ranged between 3.4% and 25% prenatally, and between 2.4% and 51% postpartum (Philpott, 2019). We suggest that all new parents be screened for depression and anxiety on a routine basis.

Not all depressed people experience extreme sadness. Often, especially in men, depression may be felt as irritability, aggression, and hostility. They may distance themselves, find distractions to avoid the family, or "check out." This certainly contributes to relationship or marital distress. Other common symptoms may be difficulty falling or staying asleep, appetite changes, racing thoughts or constant worry, and lack of joy or pleasure in things that used to be enjoyed. Some people feel helpless and hopeless. Having a new baby and an increased financial burden can really contribute to a feeling of being trapped. Being depressed is like having foggy glasses on. Everything you see gets filtered through the lenses and gets distorted. Only the negative things get through.

Depression in dads and partners also affects infant and childhood behavioral and emotional development (for details, refer to "Why Is Treatment Necessary?" in Chapter 7).

What can you do? Get support for yourself. Get educated. Find a professional trained specifically in perinatal mood and anxiety disorders. Talk to your partner, friends, or family, if you think they will listen with care. It is critical to find nonjudgmental support. Getting the help you need is a sign of strength.

To find a number of websites devoted to dad support, see the Resources section.

Things to Keep in Mind

- *You didn't cause her illness and you can't take it away.*
  Perinatal depression and anxiety are diagnosable disorders. It's no one's fault. When her brain chemistry returns to normal, she will feel like herself again.

- *She doesn't expect you to "fix it."*
  Many partners feel frustrated because they feel inadequate or unable to fix the problem. She doesn't need you to try to take the problem away. This isn't like a leaky faucet that can be repaired with a new washer.

Don't suggest quick-fix solutions. This isn't that kind of problem. She needs you to listen.

- *Get the support you need so you can be there for her.*
  We frequently see the partner becoming depressed during or after the wife's illness. You can avoid this by taking care of yourself and getting your own support from friends, family, or professionals. You should make sure to get breaks from taking care of your family. Regular exercise or other stress-reducing activity is important so you can remain a solid support. Suggest a stand-in support person while you're gone.

- *Don't take it personally.*
  Irritability and anger are common with perinatal depression/anxiety. Don't allow yourself to become a verbal punching bag. It's not good for anyone concerned. She feels guilty after saying hurtful things to you. If you feel you didn't deserve to be snapped at, explain that to her calmly.

- *Just being there with and for her is doing a great deal.*
  Being present and letting her know you support her is often all she'll need. Ask her what words she needs to hear for reassurance, and say them to her often.

- *Have realistic expectations.*
  Even a nondepressed postpartum woman cannot realistically be expected to cook dinner, clean house, and care for the baby. She might feel guilty about not measuring up to her own expectations and worry that you will also be disappointed. Remind her that parenting your child and taking care of your home is also your job, not just hers. With help from a perinatal provider your relationship and family will emerge from this crisis stronger than ever. Very often there will be

good days and bad days. Gradually, the frequency and severity of bad days will decrease. Don't assume, though, that after a few good days she is "cured." It may be a while before she is consistently having good days.

- *Let her sleep at night.*
She needs at least six hours of uninterrupted sleep per night for brain health. If you want your wife back quicker, be on duty during this time without disturbing her. Many dads and partners have expressed how much closer they are to their children because of nighttime caretaking. If you can't be up with the baby during the night, find someone who can take your place. A temporary caretaker will be worth his or her weight in gold.

- *Be on her team.*
Point out when you see improvement, like, "You're smiling more" or, "You're calling your friends again." If you don't see her improving over time, gently express your concerns and offer to accompany her to her next provider appointment.

What to Say, What Not to Say

Say:

- *We will get through this.*
- *I'm here for you.*
- *I'm on your team.*
- *I won't leave you—we're here for each other through thick and thin.*
- *I know you'll get well.*
- *If there is something I can do to help you, please tell me.*
- *I'm sorry you're suffering. That must feel awful.*
- *I love you very much.*

- *The baby loves you very much.*
- *This is temporary.*
- *You'll get yourself back.*
- *You're doing such a good job.*
  Give specific examples such as, "You sing to her so sweetly," or, "He loves it when you tickle his feet."
- *You're a great mom.*
  Again, be specific, such as, "I love how you smile at the baby."
- *This isn't your fault. If I were ill, you wouldn't blame me, and you'd take care of me.*

Do Not Say:

- *Think about everything you have to feel happy about.*
  She already knows everything she has to feel happy about. One of the reasons she feels so guilty is that she is depressed despite these things. That's the nature of depression.
- *Just relax.*
  This suggestion usually produces the opposite effect. She is already frustrated at not being able to relax despite all the coping mechanisms that have worked in the past. Anxiety produces hormones that can cause physical reactions, such as an increased heart rate, shakiness, visual changes, shortness of breath, and muscle tension. This is not something she can just will away.
- *Snap out of it.*
  If she could, she would have already. She wouldn't wish this on anyone. A person cannot snap out of any illness.
- *Just think positively.*
  It would be lovely if recovery were that simple! The nature of this illness prevents positive thinking. Depression feels like wearing distorted lenses that filter

out positive input from the environment. Only negative, guilt-ridden interpretations of the world are perceived. This illness is keeping her from experiencing the lighter, humorous, and joyful aspects of life.

From a Dad Who's Been There

This was written by Henry, Shoshana's late husband, for Shoshana's newsletter, soon after her first depression had subsided:

You've just come home from a long day at work, hoping to find a happy home—and what you find makes you want to get back into the car and leave. Your wife is in tears, the baby is crying. The house is a mess, and forget about dinner. By now you know better than to ask how her day was. Her response is always the same. "I hate this 'mother' stuff. I don't want to be anyone's mother. I want my old life back. I want to be happy again." You shrug, go to hold the baby, and wonder why your wife is feeling this way, why she's not as happy as you are about the baby, and when she will snap out of it.

You're not alone. I lived with this scene every day for two years. Every ounce of my patience was tested, but I kept hoping that things would be "normal" again. I focused on my baby daughter, the one in the midst of this mess, and kept telling myself I'd be there for her.

Slowly, slowly, my wife recovered from the illness. Today, we have that happy home we both always wanted. Be patient and tolerant. Remember, it will get better.

Five

Family and Friends

It's painful to watch someone you love struggle or suffer. It is often confusing and difficult to understand the illness or the process of recovery. Perinatal mood and anxiety disorders are real and can be debilitating, and in severe cases, life threatening. The more educated you become, the more supportive and helpful you can be. This chapter is to support and educate you, and help you become part of the healing process.

After the birth of a baby there are many changes that occur in a household. Although siblings may understand some of these changes, they won't expect their parents' moods and behavior to be different.

Children usually notice if Mom is, or has been, crying. They will notice if Mom yells or gets angry over little things. Perhaps they will notice that she stays in bed more, doesn't have the energy to take them to the park, or laugh much lately. Maybe they see her staring blankly into space, not paying much attention to them. Children can tell this is not the parent they used to know, and they need honest, clear explanations about what is occurring.

It is crucial that the path of communication with children is open. Whenever possible the parents should talk with their children about these changes. There are several important guidelines in communicating with children about what is happening.

Communicating with Children

- Even adults are often unclear about what words like *depression* or *anxiety* mean. Instead, use descriptive words like *sad, cranky, tired, weepy, worried,* or *grouchy.*
- Reassure children often that they did not cause the illness; this is not their fault, nor could they have done anything to prevent it.
- Let them know it is not the kind of illness caused by germs. You can't catch it from anyone, nor give it to anyone.
- Let the children know that Mom/Dad is getting help—seeing a doctor or counselor, taking medicine or other treatment—and it will get better. Let them know Mom/Dad may have some good and some bad times during recovery.
- Ask the children how they want to help. Perhaps they can draw a pretty picture, leave "I love you" notes around the house, and offer to help with age-appropriate tasks.
- Tell the truth. Children know if a parent is not "themself," so don't tell them everything is fine when it is not. Be direct and honest too. For instance, when it is apparent that there is sadness, say so. Sadness is just a feeling; it does not have to be logical or rational. Feelings are part of being human. To hide sadness (for example, saying, "Oh, these are happy tears"), gives the message that it is not okay to be sad.

Showing feelings teaches children how to express themselves in appropriate ways. This will not damage them. On the contrary, it can model behavior that will serve them well in the future. And by getting help you show your children that when there is something wrong, you can do something about it.

Here is an example of what a parent could say:

You may have noticed I have been crying and getting mad a lot lately. Some of the chemicals in my body are not working right, and it has been affecting how I feel and how I act. I want you to know I love you very much, and I love the baby, too. I also want you to know that this is not your or anybody else's fault. I am taking good care of myself and getting help so I can get better as fast as I can. I am probably going to have good times and bad times, but I will get better and better until I'm completely well. I am looking forward to taking you to the park again. I love you very much.

How family and friends react to the new parent's depression can critically affect recovery.

Sometimes a depressed or anxious mother feels too scared to tell her partner about uncomfortable thoughts or feelings, fearing disapproval and rejection. This mom may open up to you first, if given an opportunity. But even if she is talking openly with her partner, having the right kinds of support from her parents, in-laws, grandparents, siblings, and friends will provide her with the best environment for recovery.

When women become mothers, even if they aren't depressed, they often crave the company and approval of their own mothers. If a woman's own mother is deceased, or if their relationship is strained, it will be extra important to have another woman who can help fill that void. Because depressed mothers are, in general, even more vulnerable than nondepressed mothers, they will need extra reassurance from those around them, especially from adult females.

New moms in general are sensitive to criticism. Moms with perinatal mood and anxiety disorders are typically even more sensitive. Compliment the new mom frequently on her mothering. Avoid negative comments and unsolicited advice, especially those related to parenting.

Things to Keep in Mind

You will not be able to cure her.

You may feel frustrated that perinatal illnesses cannot be cured in the same way as other conditions. The course of this illness, even with excellent treatment, is different from that of an ear infection, for example. Where most common conditions get steadily better until they disappear, recovery during this time can be up and down.

Typically the woman advances two steps forward and feels better, and then drops one step back and "dips." She may feel hopeless when these dips occur, since depression robs her of a perspective that she is getting well. She may voice that she is back to square one and that she is not getting better.

It is important that you remind her that the dip is only temporary, she is getting better, and her moods will get back on track. A dip is not a step backward—it is simply part of the process. Over time the dips are shorter and not as deep, and the good times increase. Remind her that as long as she is going in the right direction overall, that is what is most important.

Encourage, do not insist.

Women suffering from these illnesses often feel incapable of finding the words to communicate their feelings. Let her know you are willing to listen without judgment. Trust that she will open up when she is ready. Even just being there in total silence together can be a great support. Your presence alone is tremendously helpful, even if she cannot or chooses not to speak.

Stay in the here and now.

With her up-and-down moods, the recovering woman cannot trust that the good times will last. She never knows when her moods will shift. She may be reluctant to share the good times with you for fear that you'll think she no longer needs your support. Eventually the good times will last and the dips will go away, but this process can take a while and varies greatly from person to person. Reassure her that you understand she will be riding some waves of mood for a while, and that your support won't be suddenly yanked away.

Don't let looks fool you.

Perinatal mood and anxiety disorders are often hidden illnesses. Sufferers frequently appear normal to the outside world. They can be dressed beautifully, and even with a smile, and still be deeply depressed or anxious at the same time.

Sometimes the person who is suffering might overcompensate. For instance, if there is shame, they may try to act perky in order to hide their true feelings. It is important to ask all new parents how they are doing and never assume based on appearance. So if you hear another family member say, "But she/he doesn't look depressed," you can teach them that looks can be quite deceiving when it comes to perinatal illness.

What to Say, What Not to Say

Say:

- *I'm here for you.*
- *I'm sorry you are suffering. That must feel awful.*
- *You're doing the best you can.*
- *You will get well.*
- *Would you like me to...* (insert task such as, *do the dishes or laundry*)?

- *I went through this too.*
  Only if you truly did—remember, this is not Baby Blues. If it's not true, don't say it.

Do Not Say:

- *Just buck up and tough it out.*
  Not getting adequate treatment puts sufferers at risk of chronic illness and relapse.
- *I don't get what the big deal is.*
  Depression makes everything feel like a big deal. She's overwhelmed and unable to cope. Even small chores may seem too difficult.
- *You have so much to be happy about.*
  She knows that already. She feels guilty that she is still depressed despite those things.
- *You just need more sleep.*
  Sleep is important, but is usually not all that is required to be well.
- *You just need a break from your baby.*
  Breaks are crucial, but usually they are not all that is needed.
- *I went through this too.*
  Remember, this is not Baby Blues. Don't minimize the experience by saying you've "been there" unless you really have suffered with this illness.
- *Women have been having babies for centuries.*
  And a certain percentage has been getting depressed for centuries!

What You Can Do to Help

- Prepare meals.
- Watch the baby (or other children).
- Do the laundry.

- Do the dishes.
- Sit and listen.
- Clean the house.
- Take a walk together.
- Go shopping or do errands.
- Write thank you notes.
- Be on duty at night so the parent(s) can sleep.

Six

Practitioners

All providers who touch the lives of patients during pregnancy and postpartum need this information. The fact that you are reading this book clearly indicates that you are a caring and concerned professional. Your guidance during this critical time will significantly impact the mental and physical well-being of those with perinatal mood disorders. It is important not to underreact or overreact to these symptoms. Just treat them as matter-of-factly as you would any other common perinatal experience, for example, gestational diabetes.

This chapter contains answers to the questions that we have been asked most frequently throughout the years regarding signs, symptoms, and treatment. Because a distressed parent's contact with a professional office includes the receptionist and nursing staff, it is imperative that the entire staff be knowledgeable about the information in this book.

Please remember that warning signs of distress are not always obvious for a variety of reasons. Shame, guilt, or fear of judgment may cause the woman to hide her feelings. She may present more "socially acceptable" complaints such as fatigue, headache, marital problems, or a fussy baby. Just because a woman is smiling or well groomed, don't assume that she feels good. These are hidden illnesses. Although there are risk factors to help predict PMADs, there is no particular "type" of person who becomes ill. Studies have shown that standardized screening improves detection. In England, all new mothers are screened with the Edinburgh Postnatal Depression Scale. Many states in the U.S. now have mandated screening for PMADs. The American College of Obstetricians and Gynecologists, the American Academy of Pediatrics, and the American

Association of Family Practice have all recommended perinatal screening (see the "Screening" section for more information).

We appreciate that you may be apprehensive about asking questions that might elicit strong emotions. She might feel accused of being a bad mom and become defensive. But once she hears your matter-of-fact tone, and understands no shame should be attached to issues of mental health, she likely will be able to accept the information. She'll "get" that the brain is part of the body that deserves help when needed. In the long run, you will be saving yourself time while providing quality care.

Culture and Language

Although the prevalence of perinatal mood and anxiety disorders appears to be generally the same throughout the world, reactions to these disorders vary among cultures. Where shame is a great personal threat, for example, women may be more reluctant to discuss their symptoms and will require considerable reassurance.

It's critical to take into account that nonverbal communication varies among cultures as well. For instance, a nod or a smile could signify understanding or simply respect for authority. It is also important to make clear what your role is in order to avoid unrealistic expectations.

Sociocultural factors and literacy levels should be considered when taking a medical history or completing an assessment. The perception of stress and types of stressors, as well as coping styles, differ across cultures. These will affect the patient's response to recommendations regarding which treatment methods to use or to avoid.

The level of simplicity or sophistication you use should be attuned to that of the patient, but do not assume that an educated person will automatically understand the condition better than someone with less education. For instance, avoid raising questions of self-diagnosis, such as, "Do you think you have postpartum depression?" even when a patient is highly educated. There may be an inaccurate preconceived idea of what that term means. Instead, ask specific questions about mood and behavior, which will elicit this information. These questions are outlined later in this chapter.

What to Say, What Not to Say

Say:

- *These feelings are quite common.*
- *This is treatable.*
- *You will get well.*
- *Here is some information that will help you.*

Do Not Say:

- *This is normal.*
  Depression and anxiety, while common, are not normal.
- *Join a new moms' group.*
  If a mother is clinically depressed or anxious, this may be a damaging suggestion, depending largely on the leader of the group. A depressed mother is already feeling different and inadequate compared to other new mothers. Attending a "normal" new mothers' group may intensify her alienation.

  If you know that the leader of the group is sensitive (such as those reading this book) and discusses mood problems, this mom will be fine in such a group. Ideally, she should join a group specifically designed for mothers with postpartum depression and anxiety (see Resources section). Many of our clients belong to both types of groups—one to discuss the normal new mom stuff and the other to openly express more difficult feelings.

- *Take a vacation.*
  Although a change of scenery may be nice, the depressed mother takes her brain chemistry with her. Her anxiety and depression level may actually increase due to the financial investment and disappointment that the trip did not "cure" her.

- *Just get some exercise.*
  Most depressed parents are feeling overwhelmed. Some have barely enough energy to wash a bottle or take a shower, let alone work out. For most, exercise alone will not cure depression. When she's able to take a short walk, encourage her to do so. But, until then, this is just another setup for failure.

- *Do something nice for yourself.*
  This is always a good thing, but again, it will not be enough to regulate the brain chemicals. This suggestion should be used only as part of a much larger treatment plan, and not presented as a quick fix.

- *Sleep when the baby sleeps.*
  Even a nondepressed parent may have difficulty sleeping when the baby naps during the day. Especially for those with high levels of anxiety, this might be impossible. What is most important is that she sleeps at night when the baby sleeps.

Screening

We recommend using standardized screening tools specifically designed and validated for perinatal use, such as the Edinburgh Postnatal Depression Scale (EPDS) (Cox, 2014). The EPDS has been translated into over 70 languages and is used worldwide. General depression screens are also used, including the Patient

Health Questionnaire (PHQ-9), which has been validated for perinatal use (Sidebottom, 2012). The use of the PHQ-9 is increasing, and many healthcare providers are familiar with it. For your immediate use, we have outlined informal screening questions. We use the term *perinatal psychotherapist* to indicate a psychotherapist who has had advanced training and specializes in the field of perinatal mood and anxiety disorders.

Prenatal Screening

Several prenatal screening inventories have been developed. They are listed in the Resources section. If time is too limited to use screening questionnaires, the questions in the Pre-pregnancy and Pregnancy Risk Assessment should be asked. At the bare minimum, the questions associated with the highest measure of risk, noted with an asterisk (*), must be asked. These are the questions relating to personal/family history of mental illness, previous PMAD, and severe premenstrual mood changes.

Prenatal screening using the EPDS or the PHQ-9 has been found to effectively identify mothers and fathers having symptoms of prenatal depression and anxiety. These symptoms require treatment and put them at higher risk for a postpartum mood or anxiety disorder.

Pre-pregnancy and Pregnancy Risk Assessment

Warning Signs
- Missed appointments
- Excessive worrying (about their own health or the health of the fetus)
- Looking unusually tired
- Crying
- Significant weight gain or loss

- Physical complaints with no apparent cause
- Flashbacks, fear, or nightmares regarding previous trauma
- Concern about not being a good parent

Questions to Ask

Note: Even if your clients/patients have previously experienced these disorders, they may not be aware of this fact if they were never formally diagnosed. You may need to ask about their experience with the symptoms of the disorders as opposed to using diagnostic terms in order to adequately assess.

If the answer is "yes" to any of the questions below, there is an increased risk of a PMAD.

Have you ever had episodes of being down or sad, extreme worry, repetitive thoughts or behaviors that are troublesome, extreme mood swings, loss of touch with reality, or an eating disorder?

Those with a personal history of mood or anxiety disorders need to be educated about their high risk for a perinatal episode. They should be referred to a perinatal psychotherapist to help them develop a plan of action to minimize their risk. Those with a history of bipolar disorder (very often undiagnosed) or psychosis should also be referred to a psychiatrist for a medication evaluation and observation during pregnancy and postpartum.

Are you taking any medications (prescription or nonprescription), vitamins, or herbs on a regular basis? Are you using cannabis (marijuana) or any street drugs?

Patients who are self-medicating for insomnia, anxiety, sadness, or other symptoms that may indicate a mood disorder should be evaluated by a perinatal psychotherapist. Some use caffeine, cigarettes, marijuana, herbs, alcohol, and drugs to ease emotional pain.

Have you had a previous pregnancy or postpartum mood or anxiety disorder?

Anyone answering "yes" to this question is at extremely high risk for another PMAD. They should be referred to a perinatal psychotherapist who can help them develop a plan of action to prevent or at least minimize the risk of another occurrence.

Have you ever taken any medication for depression or anxiety or mood problems?

If so, educate them about their risk of developing a perinatal mood or anxiety disorder. Observe them carefully during pregnancy and postpartum. If they are currently symptomatic, a referral for a consultation with a perinatal psychiatrist may be appropriate.

Have you ever had severe premenstrual mood changes (PMS or PMDD)?

Women whose moods are affected negatively by hormone changes are clearly at high risk during pregnancy and postpartum since there are dramatic hormonal shifts. Educate them about their risk, and follow them carefully during pregnancy and postpartum.

Do you have any family history of mental illness (undiagnosed or diagnosed), psychiatric hospitalization, or attempted suicide?

If "yes," educate them about their risk, and follow them during pregnancy and postpartum.

Postpartum Screening

A number of validated postpartum depression screening inventories are available. Most of them can easily be completed in a waiting room either electronically or in person. They can also be completed by phone, on an app, or online. The Edinburgh Postnatal Depression Screening Scale (EPDS) and the PHQ-9 are available free online.

The EPDS was developed in 1987 in Britain by Dr. John Cox, et al. It is a ten-question self-report screening tool. It has been translated into many languages and is used all over the world. It has also been effective with teens and dads. It can be found on many online sites. This tool also comes in a shortened three-question version.

In 2002 Dr. Cheryl Beck developed the Postpartum Depression Screening Scale (PDSS). It has been found to accurately screen for both postpartum depression and anxiety. The PDSS can be administered in either a short or long format. The total score can be broken down into seven symptom content scales when the long format is used. An elevated score in a particular symptom area indicates a greater amount of distress than average. The symptom scales are

- Sleeping/Eating Disturbances
- Anxiety/Insecurity
- Emotional Lability (mood swings)
- Mental Confusion
- Loss of Self, Guilt/Shame
- Suicidal Thoughts

The PDSS is more likely to identify women with symptoms of sleep disturbance, mental confusion, and anxiety.

The PHQ-9, while originally designed for use in family practice medicine to screen for depression, is now widely used in perinatal and pediatric settings. It's been validated for use in maternal and paternal depression and is available in over 30 languages.

Cutoff scores for screening may vary based on the culture of those being screened. Some cultural groups are less likely to admit potentially negative feelings or distress.

Postpartum Risk Assessment

With your postpartum patients who were not screened prenatally, ask the first six questions from the Pre-pregnancy and Pregnancy Risk Assessment (the questions marked with *), as well as those from the Postpartum Risk Assessment.

Warning Signs

- Missed appointments
- Excessive worrying (often about their health or the health of the baby)
- Looking unusually tired
- Requiring a support person to accompany her to appointments
- Significant weight gain or loss
- Physical complaints with no apparent cause
- Poor milk production or breastfeeding problems (could indicate thyroid dysfunction or a PMAD)
- Evading questions about their own well-being
- Crying
- Not willing to hold the baby or unusual discomfort handling or responding to the baby
- Not willing to allow others to care for the baby
- Excessive concern about the baby despite reassurance (for example, eating sufficiently, development, weight gain)

- Rigidity or obsessiveness (for example, regarding the baby's feeding or sleeping schedules)
- Excessive concern about appearance
- Expressing that the baby doesn't like her or that she's not a good mother
- Expressing lack of partner support

Warning Signs in the Baby

- Excessive weight gain or loss
- Delayed cognitive or language development
- Decreased responsiveness

Questions to Ask

- *How are you doing?*
  Have good eye contact while you ask this question.
- *How are you feeling about being a parent?*
  Parents who feel like they're doing a bad job or who generally don't like parenting may be depressed.
- *Do you have any particular concerns?*
- *How are you sleeping at night (quality and quantity)?*
  Six hours of uninterrupted sleep per night are required for clear thinking and functioning.
- *Can you fall asleep and stay asleep at night when everyone else is asleep?*
  Sleep problems are common with every mood and anxiety disorder. Feeling too energetic and with less perceived need for sleep may indicate a bipolar disorder.
- *How is the baby sleeping?*
  Poor infant sleep is associated with maternal depression and anxiety.
- *Who gets up at night with the baby?*
- *Who sleeps with you?* Are there other things causing sleep disruption, like snoring or pets?
- *Have you had any unusual or scary thoughts?*

If "yes," refer to a perinatal psychotherapist or psychiatrist for immediate evaluation. Some thoughts may be normal; however, others may indicate obsessive-compulsive disorder (less urgent) or psychosis (emergency).

- *Are you receiving adequate physical and emotional help?*
  A good support system of family and friends can make a significant difference.
- *Do you generally feel like yourself?*
  Parents with PMADs often report not feeling like their usual selves.
- *How is your appetite?*
  A significant change in appetite is a warning sign. Check for rapid weight loss or gain.
- *What and how often are you eating and drinking?*
  See the "Eating" section in Chapter 3.
- *If breastfeeding or pumping, how is it going?*
  Poor milk production may indicate a thyroid dysfunction or be a result of anxiety.
- *If feeding with formula, how quickly did you wean the baby?*
  Abrupt weaning can precipitate a PMAD.
- *When was your last period?*
  First menses after delivery can be a precipitating factor.
- *Are you taking any medications or herbs?*
  Self-treating for insomnia, anxiety, sadness, fatigue, or other symptoms that may indicate a mood or anxiety disorder should be evaluated by a perinatal psychotherapist.
- *Are you feeling moodier than normal (tearful, irritable, or worried)?*

This is common in mood disorders. Refer to Chapter 2 for a more complete list of symptoms.

- *Have there been any health problems for you or the baby?*

  These factors increase the risk for mood and anxiety disorders.

- *How are you feeling toward your baby?*

  Not feeling close or connected or feeling anger are examples of feelings that may indicate postpartum depression. Discomfort around the baby may indicate anxiety or OCD. Paranoia, delusions, and/or hallucinations likely indicate psychosis, which is a psychiatric emergency.

Psychotherapists, Psychologists, Social Workers

As a mental healthcare provider you may have had a relationship with the woman or couple before a pregnancy. You are a critical element in creating and being a part of the preconception planning and perinatal safety net. It is essential that you are familiar with risk factors and the most current information on how to reduce risk factors. Be familiar with the research regarding psychotherapy, relapse, and current medication recommendations. You can help monitor symptoms and work with other healthcare providers involved. Have the information in the Resources section available for all new parents and their providers.

Primary Care Providers

As a primary care provider, you may have a longstanding relationship with your patient. You have a good sense of her mental and physical health history. This puts you in an advantageous position to evaluate pre-pregnancy risk, and provide appropriate direction. Your office provides a safe haven should a pregnancy or postpartum mood problem arise. Please have information from the Resources section available, as well as referrals to local professionals trained in perinatal mood and anxiety disorders.

A woman taking psychotropic medications who is pregnant or planning a pregnancy should be encouraged to consult a psychiatrist or other prescriber specializing in perinatal disorders. Recommendations will differ based on each patient's history. Those on medication for a bipolar disorder or psychosis should be referred to a perinatal specialist to develop a medication plan. Careful monitoring throughout pregnancy and postpartum is needed to reduce the risk of illness. If a perinatal specialist is not available, you as the prescriber can directly access and consult with a specialist listed in our Resources section under Postpartum Support International.

Pediatricians and Neonatologists

Parents seek your advice for their children's well-being in all areas. Your words are powerful. While the focus of the pediatric visit is the baby, it is well documented that the mental health of the parents has a tremendous impact on the development of the children.

It's been shown that mothers with depression or anxiety breastfeed or pump for shorter durations (Pope, 2016). Mothers on medication feed their babies breast milk for a longer duration than those untreated (Grzeskowiak, 2014). Support the mom if she wishes to feed her baby breast milk while taking an antidepressant.

Parents with babies in intensive care are at high risk for depression and anxiety. They need extra support and screening. Have referrals to local professionals trained in PMADs and information in the Resources section available.

Parents should be assessed throughout the first year at well-child visits. We recommend you use a standardized postpartum screening tool.

Parents already on medication, or those who you assess need an evaluation, should be referred to a prescriber specializing in PMADs.

OB/GYNs, Midwives, and Other Women's Healthcare Providers

Your office has been a source of comfort and advice throughout the pregnancy. This intimate relationship makes it likely that a woman experiencing distress will come to you for help. However, many women will not be forthcoming with negative feelings or concerns unless specifically asked. Those with a past or present neonatal loss need monitoring and extra support. Have referrals to local professionals trained in PMADs and information in the Resources section available. Please follow up on a regular basis.

A woman taking psychotropic medication who is pregnant or planning a pregnancy should be encouraged to consult a perinatal prescriber to create a medication plan.

We recommend you use a standardized postpartum screening tool. Parents should be assessed throughout the first year. If your last appointment is before one year postpartum, make sure there is referral information available if needed at a later time.

Women already on medication, or those who you assess need a medical evaluation, should be referred to a prescriber specializing in PMADs.

Psychiatrists and Other Psychiatric Prescribers

Since you are the professionals who work most closely with psychotropic medications, many perinatal women will be referred to you for assessment and treatment of PMADs. You play an integral role in this treatment team.

Research findings and recommendations about medications in pregnancy and lactation are constantly changing. There have been some important findings recently in the area of managing medication for perinatal mood and anxiety disorders. If you are only providing medication management, make sure you give your patients the name of a psychotherapist trained in PMADs. It is essential to have a list of local resources and referrals.

Birth Doulas

Studies show that the use of a doula contributes significantly to the reduction of postpartum depression and anxiety (Falconi, 2022). As a birth doula, you are in a unique position to screen prenatally for risk and to watch for early warning signs of emotional problems. If, for instance, when administering the Pre-pregnancy and Pregnancy Risk Assessment, you discover the woman has suffered a traumatic delivery, neonatal loss, or sexual abuse, she may experience flashbacks. Have referrals to local professionals trained in perinatal mood disorders and information in the Resources section available.

A woman taking psychotropic medication who is pregnant or planning a pregnancy should be encouraged to consult a prescriber specializing in PMADs. Recommendations will differ based on each woman's history. Women on medication for a bipolar disorder or psychosis should be referred to a prescriber specializing in PMADs to develop a medication plan. These women need careful monitoring throughout pregnancy and postpartum because the risk of relapse is high, even if on medication.

Ask her if she has any particular concerns about birthing or postpartum. She then may share some information which could give you clues about her mental health. Let the woman know that one of your strengths is sensitivity to the various emotions that can occur during birth and postpartum.

Use the Pre-pregnancy and Pregnancy Risk Assessment for *all* of your clients. If you continue to see clients postpartum, use the Postpartum Risk Assessment. Keep in mind that this information can be gathered quite informally, simply through chatting. Be familiar with the questions and the pertinent information you need in order to screen.

Postpartum Doulas , Visiting Nurses, and Home Visitors

You have the opportunity to observe the home and social environments of the family, which can give crucial information about the mother's well-being and that of the family unit. For instance, if you notice a lack of partner support or signs of marital conflict, she is at greater risk for a PMAD. If her house is unusually neat and clean, ask who is doing the housework. If she is, for example, compulsively cleaning or awake in the middle of the night vacuuming, this is not normal.

Help create a healing and supportive environment, such as opening curtains to let in light, checking to see if there is healthful food, and eliminating unnecessary noise to make the home calmer and more soothing.

If you are just meeting postpartum and have not had the opportunity to screen them prenatally, we recommend you use a standardized postpartum screening tool such as the EPDS or PHQ-9. Parents should be assessed throughout the first year.

Women already on medication, or those who you assess need a medical evaluation, should be referred to a prescriber specializing in PMADs. Have referrals to local professionals trained in PMADs and information in the Resources section available.

Lactation Consultants

The role of a lactation consultant may superficially appear to be one-dimensional and relate only to the mechanics of breastfeeding. However, as we know, you are also providing tremendous emotional support. You may be the first professional to see the mother and baby during the initial postpartum weeks.

Your intimate relationship with the mother at this vulnerable time allows you to observe and listen for potential emotional problems. Postpartum moms listen carefully to what you advise and are quite trusting of you. It is so important that you help each woman decide what is right for her.

If her physical or emotional health is declining, it is obviously not good for the baby. You have a great deal of influence as to whether new mothers give themselves permission to take care of themselves (for instance, six hours of uninterrupted sleep at night, at least a few nights per week). A support person will need to feed the baby during this half of the night. Women who are suffering with depression and anxiety give up breastfeeding more quickly. When their mental health improves, it often lengthens the duration of their breastfeeding.

Sudden weaning can precipitate a mood or anxiety disorder, especially when a woman is predisposed. If she is already suffering, abrupt weaning can greatly worsen her symptoms. In addition, if a woman is depressed, there can be a great amount of guilt if at any point she decides to discontinue breastfeeding. What you say or do not say at that time can make a big difference regarding how she feels about herself.

Many professionals are unaware of the current research regarding psychotropic medications and breast milk. It is important that you are informed so you can advocate for women who need to start or continue taking medication. There are websites and apps available with this information. Have referrals to local specialists trained in PMADs and information in the Resources section available, including a professional who has experience prescribing medication during lactation.

We recommend you screen all parents using a standardized tool such as the EPDS or PHQ-9, but informal screening questions in this book can work beautifully too.

Childbirth Educators

So often we hear the lament, "Why didn't anyone warn us in our birthing classes about mood and anxiety problems during and after pregnancy?" Even though your primary focus is on labor and delivery, you have a responsibility and opportunity to educate couples about PMADs. This might be a difficult topic to discuss since no woman wants to think it could happen to her, which makes it even more important for you to initiate this conversation.

If you know a professional who is an expert in this field, you can invite her or him to speak to your class. If not, bring the subject up in a matter-of-fact manner, the same way you would any other common pregnancy or postpartum experience. Consider showing Postpartum Support International's 13-minute DVD, *Healthy Mom, Happy Family* (postpartum.net).

We can assume some of the participants in your classes are already suffering or are at risk for a PMAD. Your participants may not bring up this topic, so you need to. There is no danger in giving information, and there is great danger in omitting it. Her partner might soak up this information even if the mother-to-be does not. It is often the spouse who later recognizes the symptoms and realizes he or his wife may need help.

Hand out some information from the Resources section and the name and number of a professional trained in PMADs.

If you follow up with participants, ask about their feelings regarding the challenges as well as the joys of parenthood. Be sure to call participants who you have not been in touch with since the classes. They may not be doing well and could be trying to avoid an uncomfortable situation.

New Parent Group Leaders

If there are ten women in your group, remember that, statistically, one or two of them will have a PMAD. Rarely will this woman be brave enough to disclose her feelings, since she will most likely be experiencing guilt and shame. She will be aching for someone to open the door to this discussion and give her permission to express how she is really feeling. If partners are present, ask them how they themselves are doing. Dads/partners may have preexisting mood or anxiety disorders. The stress of a pregnancy can also worsen symptoms. No matter what, dads and partners need and deserve support too.

Encourage discussion about the normal feelings accompanying adjustment to parenting and the relationship to oneself, partner, baby, friends, and family. You can easily work in some facts about moods and behaviors that fall outside the realm of normal adjustment.

For each new group, make sure this topic gets explored in a nonjudgmental manner. If you prefer, you can invite a professional with expertise to lead a discussion. In any case, use the information in the Resources section and the names and numbers of local professionals trained in PMADs. Consider showing Postpartum Support International's 13-minute DVD, *Healthy Mom, Happy Family.*

Adjunct Professionals

There are many other wonderful professionals who touch the lives of pregnant and postpartum parents. For example, physical therapists and instructors in prenatal and postpartum exercise should mention the possibility of mood and anxiety disorders, since you are encountering suffering women all the time. Above all, making the information in the Resources section available will support the pregnant and postpartum parents with whom you work.

Seven

Treatment

Why Is Treatment Necessary?

Science evolves and changes our beliefs and views. We used to believe that babies should sleep on their stomachs. Now we know that putting babies to sleep on their backs reduces the risk of sudden infant death syndrome (SIDS). Research about perinatal mood and anxiety disorders has also taught us new things. In the past, people thought these illnesses didn't exist, or if they did, women didn't need treatment. It was thought that women should suffer through them and wait to recover on their own. We now know how incorrect and harmful that thinking was. Untreated illness in pregnancy will most likely lead to postpartum illness, and all the while everyone involved is negatively affected. Untreated mood and anxiety disorders may (or may not) go away after a time, and increase the likelihood of another episode later in life. Most people, if diagnosed with diabetes or cancer, would immediately seek treatment. Perinatal illnesses are no different—they require treatment and care.

Untreated mood and anxiety illnesses in pregnancy are associated with (Meltzer-Brody, 2014; Rada 2021):

- Self-medication with potentially unsafe over-the-counter remedies, tobacco, alcohol, or marijuana and other drugs
- Poor nutrition and lack of self-care
- Appetite changes and abnormal weight gain or loss
- Poor fetal growth and low birth weight
- Premature birth (less than 37 weeks)
- Babies who cry more and are more difficult to soothe and calm

89

- Behavioral problems in preschoolers
- Developmental delays in toddlers
- Antisocial, aggressive, and violent behavior in teens

Moms who have *untreated* postpartum illness may:

- Have babies whose brain waves show depression
- Have difficulty with bonding and attachment
- Breastfeed for shorter duration
- Have babies who cry more
- Have children with poor language and cognitive (thinking) development and poor school readiness
- Be less likely to use car seats and are more likely to use harsh discipline
- Be less likely to start feeding with breast milk and less likely to continue
- Have children who are 50% more likely to suffer anxiety or depression when they become teens

When Dads Have Depression

According to a study by Ramchandani in 2008, 3½-year-olds were found to have problems—boys more than girls. Four-year-old children of fathers with major depression were more likely to have been treated by professionals for speech, language, and behavioral problems. Depression in fathers is significantly associated with psychiatric disorders in their children seven years later—in particular, disruptive behavioral problems in boys.

It's also been shown that treating depression or anxiety in parents is not always enough to repair the mother-infant or mother-child attachment and relationship. Special attention needs to be given to these relationships in the healing process. Activities that involve physical touch, such as infant massage, have been shown to be helpful. Professionals who work in this field include developmental psychologists and infant mental health specialists.

Untreated illness affects the whole family. You need and deserve to be well!

Research

Research doesn't always tell the whole story. There are lots of challenges understanding research. Here are some questions to ask:

Where is it reported?

The Internet is often not a reliable source. Forums and blogs frequently yet inaccurately interpret scientific studies (we recommend those listed in the Resources section). Often they contain individuals' personal stories. Even large well-respected news sources blur scientific conclusions to create attention-getting headlines.

How many people were studied?

The smaller the study population, the less meaningful the result. The most valuable studies have thousands of participants, or at least other research that repeats the results of the smaller study.

What was measured or studied? How was it measured?

For example, there are many studies on the effects of medication on the fetus. Some studies base results on prescriptions written, and then look at the infants. The problem? Just having a prescription, even if filled, does not always mean the woman actually took the medication. And even if she took the medication, she may not have taken the dose prescribed or necessary to treat her depression or anxiety.

Many studies that looked at the impact of medications on a fetus have not taken into account other critical factors that can impact outcomes, like cigarettes, drugs, alcohol, poor nutrition, or the effects of depression or anxiety if the woman was on an inadequate dose of medication. Genetic risk is also important to consider, for instance, when looking at autism.

Our goal is to translate and summarize the reliable studies to help you make the best decisions for you and your family.

Prevention

Prevention of a perinatal mood and anxiety disorder is, of course, the ultimate goal. Research is beginning to evaluate preventive methods, primarily counseling and educational programs (O'Connor, 2019). Interventions for women at the highest risk for a PMAD have been very successful in decreasing the likelihood or severity of an illness occurring. The women studied have had a history of depression, abuse, unplanned pregnancy, stressful life events, partner violence, and complications during pregnancy. What follows is some of the best information currently available.

In an older Canadian study, women at high risk for postpartum depression were offered an extended postpartum hospital stay (up to five days) in a private room. Their babies slept in the nursery at night so the moms could sleep without interruption. The moms also met once with a member of the Canadian Women's Health Concerns Clinic during their stay. This study highlighted the importance of uninterrupted sleep and support, as these women were less likely to suffer from postpartum depression, and for those who did get depressed, the depression was milder (Ross, 2005).

There are also studies showing that psychotherapy online, in person, or in groups can be used effectively for prevention of depression and anxiety. Groups utilizing interpersonal psychotherapy, cognitive behavioral therapy, and psychoeducation during pregnancy reduce the occurrence of postpartum depression and anxiety (Werner, 2015; Wagas, 2022; Zimmermann, 2023). An online program for the prevention of postpartum depression offered in English and in Spanish was also found to be effective (Barrera, 2015). Online-based prenatal services including psychotherapy, resources, and psychoeducation were found helpful in reducing PMADs (Rubin-Miller, 2023), including in young people (Ronan, 2024).

Mindfulness-based interventions including those delivered by mobile platforms are helpful for perinatal depression and anxiety (Leng, 2023).

A study of Chinese women found that those who took folic acid supplements during at least six months of their pregnancy had lower rates of postpartum depression (Yan, 2017). In a small study in the United States, it was shown that a supplement containing L-methylfolate and folic acid both prevented and treated depression in women planning to conceive or who were already pregnant. EnbraceHR is a prescription prenatal vitamin for all women, even those with MTHFR (a gene that makes it difficult to metabolize folic acid or folate) (Freeman, 2019).

An exciting study published in 2023 (Guintivano) examined genetic samples from all over the world. They found that major depression and postpartum depression may have specific genetic markers. So, genetically, some people may be at an increased risk because of heredity. A small study in China (Sheng, 2023) of women who had C-sections found that biomarkers of spinal fluid may predict PPD. In the future these findings may guide risk assessment and treatment.

New research is beginning to look at how microorganisms in a person's gastrointestinal system including many bacteria, fungi, viruses, and other organisms can contribute to perinatal mood disorders. This research may lead to both prevention and treatment (Zhang, 2023).

All new parents need a wellness plan, because all parents need nurturing. This is not a luxury—it is a necessity! Everyone who is at high risk should meet with a knowledgeable perinatal psychotherapist before pregnancy to create a prenatal and postpartum wellness plan. This plan may include follow-up appointments with other professionals, sleep arrangements, meal preparation, and getting breaks away from the baby during the week. If an illness occurs, a wellness plan will be in place that will support and speed recovery.

Information and education are critical components of treatment. Sometimes this is all that is needed to recover. It's therapeutic to know these illnesses have names and are treatable.

Psychotherapy

Psychotherapy is talk therapy. A perinatal psychotherapist is someone who has had specific training in issues related to perinatal mood and anxiety disorders, and perinatal loss. Training in general depression and anxiety is not enough to qualify the provider to treat the unique set of issues for PMADs.

Psychoeducation is an important part of perinatal therapy. Psychoeducation includes offering information and explaining issues related to perinatal illness and treatment. The psychotherapist should be familiar with local support as well as other trustworthy resources online and in print. Psychotherapy can be used with individuals, with the couple, with family members, or in a group setting.

Pregnancy and postpartum treatment involve crisis management. The treatments found to be most effective specifically for PMADs are short-term, brief psychotherapies focused on symptom reduction and an improvement in functioning. This is not the time for long-term psychodynamic or psychoanalytic therapy.

Two types or models of psychotherapy have been well studied and shown to be effective for the prevention and treatment of PMADs. These models are called Interpersonal Psychotherapy (IPT) (Sockol, 2018; Bright, 2020) and Cognitive Behavioral Therapy (CBT) (Stamou, 2018; Li, 2022). In both models the therapist plays an active role facilitating and directing discussion and teaching problem-solving skills. Psychotherapy has been shown to have a long-lasting positive impact.

CBT works by helping monitor and change thinking and behavior through education and skill building. CBT helps clients develop new ways to evaluate life experiences including trauma, and teaches practical tools that can be used immediately.

The IPT model works to help clients address role changes, transitions and conflicts, loss and grief, and build interpersonal skills as well as support resources.

Both models focus on client strengths. When unable to process or apply psychotherapeutic strategies, medication or alternative treatments are often additionally useful.

There is a small but growing amount of research on the effectiveness of Eye Movement Desensitization and Reprocessing (EMDR) for birth trauma. EMDR has been well studied in non-perinatal populations for treatment of disorders such as anxiety, depression, OCD, chronic pain, addictions, and other distressing life experiences (Maxfield, 2019). There is specific training for perinatal EMDR practitioners. We have seen this therapy help our clients recover.

Social Support

Good social support provides nonjudgmental listening, feedback, and information. It creates an environment where women can see that they are not alone or to blame, and sometimes includes specially trained people who are survivors of PMADs. Social support can be emotional support as well as practical physical support (babysitting, housecleaning, bringing meals). Support networks include support groups, telephone support, home visitors, email, text, online groups, faith/spiritual communities, family/friends.

Numerous studies have shown that a variety of social support models are effective in the prevention and recovery of PMADs (Dennis, 2013; Fang, 2022). Contact Postpartum Support International (see the Resources section) for assistance in finding social support.

Complementary and Alternative Medicine (CAM)

Studies are currently being conducted regarding treatment in pregnancy and postpartum that do not involve prescription medication. *Complementary* treatments are those used in addition to the chosen treatment(s) as enhancements. *Alternative* treatments are used instead of medication.

As always, having a correct diagnosis is essential before starting any kind of complementary or alternative treatment. For instance, just like an antidepressant, SAMe, St. John's wort, and bright light therapy can all trigger hypomania or mania in women with bipolar illness. *Natural* does not necessarily mean "safe." Be sure to talk with your healthcare provider before taking supplements or using any of these treatments.

Found Effective and Safe

Massage and Yoga

Data regarding the therapeutic effect of infant massage for both parents and babies (Dehkordi, 2019) and prenatal yoga (Battle, 2015; Villar-Alises, 2023) are beginning to emerge. A systematic review of research found that infant massage in a group setting or in the home reduced maternal depression, improved maternal sleep quality, reduced anxiety, and lessened feelings of guilt (Geary, 2023).

Exercise

Physical exercise was found to significantly reduce perinatal depressive symptoms in a multinational study (Liu, 2022). This study included yoga, walking, exercise with baby, and water exercise.

Morning Light

Morning bright light therapy (natural sunlight or a special light box) is being used either as a complementary or alternative treatment for depression (Bais, 2020; Donmez, 2022; Garbazza 2022). Studies have shown this treatment to be helpful during and after pregnancy. Although light boxes can be quite effective, they are not for everyone. Depending on your diagnosis, they can be harmful. Make sure you are working with a professional with expertise to prescribe your individual treatment.

Night Light

Researchers at John Carroll University developed special glasses that have been clinically proven with double-blind studies to naturally help nighttime sleep, and minimize bipolar mania (Esaki, 2020) and depression during pregnancy and postpartum (Bennett, 2009). When parents-to-be and new parents need to get up during the night, exposing their eyes to light can cut off the flow of melatonin, the sleep hormone. It can also upset the circadian rhythm, the "internal clock." On nights after that, the melatonin may not flow at the normal time, making it difficult to fall asleep. Over time, disruption of the circadian rhythm plus sleep deprivation can result in depression. You can find these light bulbs and glasses plus the research at LowBlueLights.com. Just as all light boxes are not created equal, beware of other "wannabe" lenses that are ineffective. Go where the research is.

Omega-3

There is some evidence about the effectiveness of omega-3 essential fatty acids in both the prevention and treatment of prenatal and postpartum depression (Sarris, 2020; Zhang 2020). The American Psychiatric Association recommends that patients with a mood disorder take 1 gm EPA (eicosapentaenoic acid) plus DHA (docosahexaenoic acid) daily. Read the labels carefully to make sure you are getting both EPA and DHA. These omega-3s are from fish oil, not the plant sources, which are different. Omega-3s are recommended as a complementary treatment. If you take omega-3s while using breast milk, the baby's neurological development may also be enhanced (these "lipophilic acids" have now been added to many baby formulas).

TMS

Repetitive transcranial magnetic stimulation (TMS) uses noninvasive brain stimulation and is showing great promise in the treatment of major depression. TMS is approved by the FDA for the treatment of major depressive disorder in adults, and studies have been conducted with depressed pregnant and postpartum women. Depression was reduced significantly within three weeks of beginning treatment, and no ill effects were seen in the moms, fetuses, or breastfeeding babies. TMS may be an effective therapy for women who choose not to go on medication (Miuli, 2023). TMS treatment often involves daily sessions for up to six weeks.

Acupuncture

A few studies have found that acupuncture is helpful treatment for mild to moderate depression in pregnancy (Manbur, 2010; Ormsby, 2020). As of now, acupuncture to treat postpartum depression has not been shown to be effective (Li, 2019).

Not Proven Effective or Safe

Marijuana

Marijuana (cannabis) is now one of the most widely used substances during pregnancy in the U.S. and Canada. Today, it is more accessible and legal in many locations. Marijuana is detectable in the placenta, amniotic fluid, and in the fetus. Prenatal use was associated with smaller babies, low birth weight and preterm births, and more Neonatal Intensive Care Unit (NICU) admissions (Shi, 2021; Marchand, 2022). Cannabis has been shown to have a negative effect on the placenta (which provides nutrients and oxygen to the growing fetus) and thus contributes to poor neonatal outcomes (Metz, 2023). The use of CBD (a component of marijuana) has also been shown to contribute to poor fetal growth. Another large study including data from over seven countries (Sorkhou, 2023) confirmed an association with low birth weight, preterm birth, and NICU admissions with marijuana use. Even with legal medical marijuana, no "safe" dose has been established for perinatal use. There are increasing concerns for the child regarding long-term brain development and behavior when exposed in utero (Jaques, 2014; Gunn, 2016; Friedrich, 2017).

The American College of Obstetricians and Gynecologists (2021) says, "Pregnant women or women contemplating pregnancy should be encouraged to discontinue use of marijuana for medicinal purposes in favor of an alternative therapy for which there are better pregnancy-specific safety data. The effects of marijuana use may be as serious as those of cigarette smoking or alcohol consumption."

Marijuana has not been well studied in breastfeeding mothers. We do know that traces of marijuana (THC and CBD) have been found in breast milk up to six days after use (Bertrand, 2018; Moss, 2021), and the amount might be even higher than that found in the mother's blood. Exposure through breast milk may affect brain development in children under one year.

If you are using marijuana on a regular basis, we encourage you to speak with your healthcare provider. Consider what you need treating and what is the safest way to treat that problem.

Herbs

Little research has been done on the safety or effectiveness of herbs during pregnancy or nursing (Deligiannidis, 2014). Herbal remedies are often produced with little or no regulation or safety monitoring. You cannot tell the quality or quantity of the active ingredient you're receiving in each dose. Because there is no governmental regulation on herbal preparations, studies have found that the measured amounts of the active ingredients vary considerably from those claimed on the labels—from 0% to 109% for capsules and from 31% to 80% for tablets. It is impossible to know what and how much of the herb you're actually taking. In addition, dangerous contaminants have been found in some herbal formulations.

There are very few studies evaluating the safety of St. John's wort (Hypericum perforatum) during pregnancy or in breast milk (Zepeda, 2023). There is no research that shows that St. John's wort is an effective treatment for anxiety or obsessive-compulsive disorder. St. John's wort interacts with a number of medications, including those for heart disease, depression, seizures, certain cancers, and birth control pills. This means St. John's wort makes the birth control pill less effective. St. John's wort should not be taken with an SSRI because they work on the same chemicals in the brain.

Placenta

There have been a number of articles reporting that eating placenta prevents postpartum blues and possibly protects against postpartum depression and anxiety. Placenta eating has been part of a few cultural rituals around the world. And, indeed, some animal species do eat the placenta after birth, but we don't know the reason or if the behavior benefits the mother. Most of the studies presented by advocates of placental encapsulation do not evaluate human ingestion and mood, energy, or hormone levels. In 2017 a study about placenta encapsulation and postpartum mood was published (Young, 2017). Unfortunately, they only studied 12 women who ingested placenta capsules and compared them to 13 women who took placebo (did not contain placenta) capsules. There was no benefit or difference for the women taking placenta capsules compared to the women who took placebos. Remember that 30% of people will feel better when given a placebo or "sugar pill."

In a larger study in 2019, there was no evidence to show that women with a history of mood disorders have any benefits in mood, energy, lactation, or vitamin B12 levels after ingesting their placenta. And a study done in 2023 (Benyshek) showed there was no evidence that placenta consumption lowers the risk of postpartum depression.

Medications for PMADs

The most immediate goal of treatment is to alleviate suffering as quickly as possible. Medication is usually started at a low dosage, and increased as rapidly as possible to whatever the effective dose is for that person. Undertreating can lead to chronic problems and suffering, and increases the risk of relapse. It has been shown repeatedly that maintenance on medications during pregnancy in women with mood disorders significantly reduces the risk of recurrence (Stevens, 2019).

What follows here are guidelines only. All treatment must be individualized. For medication management we recommend you see a prescriber with knowledge in treating perinatal illnesses. No matter what treatments you choose, someone with expertise should monitor you. Be persistent! If one practitioner or provider, or one medication or treatment method doesn't work or feel like a good fit, try another. The goal is to feel like you again. Feeling "OK" or "better" is not good enough.

The medications that are of most concern during pregnancy are the anti-epileptic (seizure) drugs used for mood stabilization. Valproic acid (Depakote) and carbamazepine (Tegretol) are known to cause birth defects and IQ problems (Andrade, 2018). If a woman on medication discovers she is pregnant, the fetus has already been exposed, and the risk of illness due to changing medications is high. The potential risks of medication must always be weighed against the long-lasting risks of illness—on the mother, fetus, infant, and family.

Quite a bit of research has been conducted regarding the use and effectiveness of certain prescription medications during pregnancy and lactation that effectively combat and treat PMADs. These prescription medications are monitored by the Food and Drug Administration (FDA) to make sure there are no contaminants, and that the dose is indeed the stated dose.

For many years the FDA used a confusing and misleading rating scale for safety labeling of medication during pregnancy. The old categories used a rating system labeling medications A, B, C, D, or X. For example, medications with less research were often labeled safer (A, B, C), while medications that often had more research were sometimes labeled less safe (D or X), regardless of the outcome of the studies. In June 2015, that old system was discarded and replaced by a more informative safety labeling of medications used during pregnancy and in breast milk.

Pregnancy and Medication

Counseling alone is enough for many, but for some, medication is necessary to reduce serious symptoms of depression and anxiety, including OCD. What we do know is that untreated illness in pregnancy is associated with poor prenatal, infant, and child outcomes. There is no increased risk of miscarriage or birth defects from antidepressants taken during pregnancy, even in the first trimester (Kjaersgaard, 2013; Eleftheriou, 2023).

Current thinking regarding the use of medications in pregnancy has evolved over the years. Researchers who have spent years investigating the potential effects of medication on the fetus have shifted their focus to the harmful effects on the fetus when mental illness goes untreated. These experts agree that maternal depression and anxiety must be evaluated and treated to maximize a positive outcome for the baby and the mother. When evaluating risks of medication in pregnancy, it is critical to remember that all normal pregnancies have around a 3% chance of a birth defect, and up to 20% of all pregnancies end in miscarriage.

Pregnancy causes changes in metabolism and blood volume; therefore, higher doses of medications may be required to achieve an adequate reduction in symptoms. One study found that in order to remain symptom-free, two-thirds of women required an increase in dosage at six and a half months into the pregnancy.

The *American Journal of Psychiatry* published an article stating that *not* prescribing antidepressants to a woman who is depressed or likely to become ill again during pregnancy may cause more risks to the mom and fetus than the risks of exposure to medication. Staying on medication for depression and bipolar disorders during pregnancy significantly reduces the risk of illness during pregnancy (Stevens, 2019).

There are many challenges when studying potential outcomes of medication during pregnancy. Studies often look at drugs prescribed, which doesn't always mean the medication was actually taken. Pregnancy outcomes can be impacted by other factors including smoking, poverty, stress levels, and how well the illness is actually treated.

Following is a summary of commonly used prescription medications for perinatal mood and anxiety disorders.

Antianxiety Medications

While the SSRIs are often used to treat anxiety, panic and OCD, it can sometimes take several weeks before a reduction in symptoms is noticed. Another group of medications, the benzodiazepines, are used for immediate relief of anxiety. Sometimes they are used with SSRIs to keep anxiety under control, usually on a short-term basis. Alprazolam (Xanax) and lorazepam (Ativan) are shorter acting (out of your system more quickly), while diazepam (Valium) and clonazepam (Klonopin) are longer acting.

In 2023 a study by Meng found that benzodiazepine use in early pregnancy increased the risk of miscarriage. There is now some evidence that maternal anxiety may itself contribute to poor outcomes such as preterm birth and low birthweight. Large literature reviews found that prenatal use of benzodiazepines was not associated with a risk of malformations (Grigoriadis, 2019; Szpunar, 2022; Chan, 2023).

Babies born exposed to high doses at the end of pregnancy may experience some temporary problems. However, anxiety or panic disorder should be treated. The lowest effective dose for the shortest period of time is recommended. It's important to speak to a reproductive prescriber if you are on benzodiazepines before (if possible) or during a pregnancy.

Antidepressants

Since we receive so many antidepressant questions from our pregnant clients (and those on medications who are considering another pregnancy), we have addressed some of the biggest concerns here. Brand names may vary by country, so we are including both brand and generic names of medications.

When compared to siblings, babies exposed to antidepressants during pregnancy had *no* increased risk of preterm births, autism spectrum disorder, small for gestational age, birth defects, attention deficit hyperactivity disorder (ADHD), behavioral problems, neurodevelopmental deficits, or lower school achievement (Besag, 2023).

Do antidepressants cause miscarriage?

In a review and analysis of over 735 studies, it was found the risk of miscarriage was the same in women with depression as women who took antidepressants for depression (Kjaersgaard, 2013). More recently another large review of studies also found no increased risk of miscarriage with antidepressants used during pregnancy (Smith, 2024).

Can antidepressants cause prematurity?

A large review of studies found insignificant differences in prematurity rates when comparing women on antidepressants to depressed women not on medication (Mitchell, 2018).

Does antidepressant use in pregnancy cause birth defects?

In all births, whether medication is present or not, there is a about a 3% chance of birth defects. It was found that antidepressant use in the first trimester was *not* associated with an increased risk of birth defects (Gao, 2018; Tak, 2017).

What about Persistent Pulmonary Hypertension of the Newborn and antidepressants?

Persistent Pulmonary Hypertension of the Newborn (PPHN) occurs in about 0.1% to 0.2% of all newborns. It is rare, but serious. It's unclear if antidepressants increase this risk because there are other known risk factors unrelated to antidepressant use such as obesity, smoking, shorter pregnancies, cesarean birth, and depression (Eleftheriou 2023).

Do antidepressants cause poor neonatal adaptation or withdrawal?

This refers to symptoms (often breathing and shaking) that are sometimes seen in newborns who were exposed to some medications during the last trimester of pregnancy. It is unclear if this is caused by too much serotonin (a brain chemical) in the baby, or a withdrawal from the medication. Reported rates vary from 10% to 30%, and seem more common in babies exposed to paroxetine (Paxil). The symptoms begin in the first few days of life, and usually are gone within 3–5 days. A joint report of The American Psychiatric Association and the American College of Obstetricians and Gynecologists notes that discontinuing medication to avoid symptoms in the newborn may lead to relapse in the mother. This is a mild syndrome that most often does not require treatment. It goes away by itself. Stopping medication in the last trimester puts a mother at greater risk of depression at the end of pregnancy and during postpartum.

Do antidepressants cause autism?

No. Several large studies have shown that antidepressants do not cause autism (Brennan, 2023; Yamamoto-Saskai, 2019; Janecka, 2018). However, maternal depression in pregnancy was found to be a significant risk factor for autism (Aldera, 2022).

Has anyone found problems in older children exposed to antidepressant medication during pregnancy?

In a study of children tested at ages 3 to 7, IQ and development tests were all normal. This included first-trimester exposure. It was found that severity of maternal depression during pregnancy predicted children's behavior problems. The use of antidepressants and the dose or length of time taken were not predictors of cognitive or behavioral problems. Another study looking at children 4 to 5 years of age found that prenatal antidepressant use was not associated with behavioral or emotional problems in early childhood. At a conference of the Pediatric Academic Societies in 2018, a study was presented evaluating prenatal exposure to SSRIs and thinking and attention skills in 12-year-olds. They found children who were exposed to medication did better with skills related to thriving in school and later in the workplace. These skills included creative problem solving, the ability to focus, attention, and self-control.

We do know that untreated illness in parents can cause long-term emotional and behavioral problems in children (Gutierrez-Galve, 2018). If you are already on an antidepressant, remember that discontinuing your medication before delivery, a time that is high risk for depression and anxiety, can put you at significant risk for illness. Speak to someone who knows the research before you make any changes in your medication. In addition, the top researchers maintain that there is no reason to change from one antidepressant to another. *Go with what works and gets the quickest results.*

In a very exciting development, the United States Food and Drug Administration (FDA) on March 19, 2019, approved a unique medication called Zulresso (brexanolone). It's the first medication specifically designed to treat postpartum depression. It requires a three-day intravenous infusion. In the study, women suffering from moderate to severe postpartum depression felt a significant relief in symptoms within 24 to 48 hours. On August 4, 2023, the FDA approved Zurzuvae (zuranolone), the first pill specifically developed and approved for treatment of postpartum depression. It is unlike other antidepressants in that it targets different brain chemicals.

In a research trial using zuranolone every evening for two weeks (Deligiannidis, 2023), mood improvement was seen as early as in three days as compared with those taking placebo pills. Side effects were few and the medication was well tolerated. At this point little research has been done about breast milk safety while taking zuranolone. LactMed, a National Institute of Health program, states that low amounts of zuranolone are passed into the breast milk and is not expected to have negative effects in infants consuming breast milk (see Resources section for more information).

Antipsychotics

These drugs are also called *major tranquilizers*. Older high-potency antipsychotics such as haloperidol (Haldol) have been recommended in the past over low-potency or atypical agents throughout pregnancy. These atypical antipsychotic medications are used to treat schizophrenia, bipolar disorder, major depression, PTSD, and anxiety disorders. Exposure to these medications is not associated with the risk of larger than normal infants, stillbirth, and miscarriage; however, these medications are associated with a very small increased risk of obstetric and neonatal problems. It is not clear yet if the increased risk is due to the medications or the underlying illness. Aripiprazole (Abilify), olanzapine (Zyprexa), and quetiapine (Seroquel) are not associated with increased risks of major birth defects or neurodevelopment problems (Straub, 2022). A large study conducted in six countries found that antipsychotic medication did not pose a risk for major birth defects (Huybrechts, 2023).

If you are considering taking one of these medications during pregnancy, please sign up with the National Pregnancy Registry for Atypical Antipsychotics (see Resources section).

Electroconvulsive Therapy (ECT)

ECT is considered an acceptable treatment for severe depression, bipolar disorder, schizophrenia, or psychosis in pregnancy (Rose, 2020). ECT is not a treatment for prenatal anxiety, panic, or obsessive-compulsive disorder (OCD).

Mood Stabilizers

Before getting pregnant, ideally, women on these medications should consult with a prescriber familiar with the latest research to plan how to best manage their illness during the course of a pregnancy. For those already pregnant, a consultation is necessary to determine the most appropriate medication plan.

Women with bipolar disorder should consider continuing on medication throughout pregnancy, because the danger of relapse is so high. In one study, 24% of women with a history of chronic bipolar disorder became ill during pregnancy even while on medication, so stopping medication is obviously quite risky. A study of bipolar women who discontinued mood stabilizers when they became pregnant found that they were twice as likely to have a relapse during the pregnancy. Within three months, half of the women relapsed, and by six months, about 70% had relapsed. Restarting medication after stopping it in the first trimester does not protect well against relapse (Viguera, 2007).

Medications used for seizure disorders such as epilepsy are often used as mood stabilizers in women with bipolar disorder. Lamotrigine (Lamictal), also an anti-seizure medication, is now considered the anti-epileptic drug of choice for pregnant women with severe bipolar depressive episodes, and may also help prevent severe postpartum depression (Wesseloo, 2017).

Lithium is an anti-mania medication used to treat bipolar disorders. In the past, lithium was believed to carry a small risk of a cardiac problem in the fetus called Ebstein's anomaly. The latest research shows that this cardiac problem is most likely related to maternal mental health problems rather than lithium (Boyle, 2017). No significant neurobehavioral or developmental problems have been reported in children who were exposed to lithium during pregnancy.

Other mood stabilizers, such as carbamazepine (Tegretol) and valproic acid (Depakote), increase the rate of neural tube defects and other birth defects. Children examined at 3 years of age were found to have decreased IQ when exposed to Tegretol during pregnancy. Because of this, an increased dose of folic acid is often used in addition to Tegretol or Depakote if either of these medications must be continued.

Sleep Aids

Depression and anxiety can cause problems falling or staying asleep. Additionally, poor sleep can contribute to mood and anxiety problems. Sleep is an essential part of the treatment plan. Cognitive behavioral therapy for insomnia (CBT-I) has been shown to be very effective during pregnancy, even when received online (Felder, 2020). Sometimes medication may be necessary, especially at the beginning of treatment. There are several over-the-counter medications that are considered fine to use while pregnant. These are doxylamine (Unisom) and diphendramamine (Benadryl).

Trazadone (Deseryl) and amitriptyline (Elavil) are antidepressants that have a sedative effect. Zolpidem (Ambien) has a faster rate of onset and is considered acceptable in pregnancy when needed (Chan, 2023).

Postpartum

On occasion the birth of a baby may bring about the need to change the medication treatment plan. A consultation with a perinatal prescriber is advised if breast milk will be used to feed the baby. Most medications are found in low levels in breast milk, and are considered very low risk to the infant. There is no one "best" medication. The medication that works best will be optimal for the baby and family.

Thyroid

Up to 16% of postpartum women will develop postpartum thyroiditis (an inflammation of the thyroid). In the early stages of thyroiditis, women may experience anxiety or depression. Sometimes this condition is temporary and will go away without treatment in about six months. But for others it can lead to chronic thyroiditis and hypothyroidism (low thyroid levels such as Hashimoto's thyroiditis).

Since thyroid disorders can cause depression and anxiety, ask your provider to check your blood. The following tests are recommended for all women with postpartum mood complaints: free T4, TSH, anti-TPO, and antithyroglobulin. It is important to check for the antithyroid antibodies (anti-TPO and antithyroglobulin) since there have been many cases where the T4 and TSH levels were within normal ranges but the antithyroid antibody levels were elevated. If thyroid labs are abnormal, we recommend an evaluation by an endocrinologist.

Hormone Therapy

It appears that it is not a low level of hormones that causes mood problems for most postpartum women. Rather, it's the shifting of hormone levels that some women are sensitive to (Shiller, 2015).

Those sensitive to hormonal shifts, including those with postpartum depression and anxiety who choose oral contraceptives (birth control pills), need to be monitored closely for mood changes. Women may experience fewer mood problems on a monophasic birth control pill as compared to a triphasic birth control pill. The monophasic pill delivers the same ratio of estrogen and progesterone, unlike the triphasic, in which the ratio changes weekly.

Women with a history of increased moodiness on oral contraceptives should consider alternate methods of contraception, as they are at an increased risk of postpartum depression (Larsen, 2023). Synthetic progesterone (progestin) including the "minipill" has been associated with a worsening of symptoms in some women. Medroxyprogesterone acetate (Depo-Provera), a long-acting progesterone injection, is not always a good option since it cannot be discontinued should it aggravate mood problems. There have also been reports of mood problems after insertion of the progesterone-releasing IUD. These mood problems usually resolve once the IUD is removed. Hormone therapy is not recommended as sole treatment for postpartum psychiatric disorders.

Medications

If you or a blood relative has had a positive experience with a particular medication for the same diagnosis, that would be the first choice. Few studies have been done on the effectiveness any one particular medication has over another in the treatment of postpartum depression/anxiety. There is not one medication that, in general, is better than the others for treating postpartum depression and anxiety. The "best" one is the one that works. In our experience all the SSRIs work well. Each woman has her own individual chemistry, which will work better with certain medications than with others. Treatment of anxiety, including obsessive-compulsive disorder, usually requires a higher dosage than that used to treat depression. The goal of treatment is to reach 100% "back to yourself." Just feeling better is not good enough. Undertreating can lead to chronic illness and increased risk of relapse.

We've worked with many clients who say that, once treated, they feel better than they have in years (or ever). They had been anxious or depressed and hadn't realized it previously.

Medications and Breast Milk

Giving a baby breast milk has great benefits for both the baby and mother. For some depressed women, breast milk may feel like the only positive thing they have to offer the baby. Most medications for depression and anxiety are found in very low amounts in breast milk and in the babies. There are, however, a few medications that are not recommended or must be used with caution.

Antianxiety Medications

Low doses of short-acting medications such as alprazolam (Xanax) or lorazepam (Ativan) are often prescribed for occasional use for anxiety, panic, and poor sleep. The National Institute of Health's LactMed database (2023) found that no adverse effects were seen in infants.

Antidepressants

It's considered safe to feed with breast milk while taking antidepressants. The first choice for every woman should be a medication that has worked for her in the past or one that has been used successfully with a blood relative.

The benefits of breast milk far outweigh any known risks of medications. Behaviorally and developmentally, these infants and children are normal.

Antipsychotics

Also called *major tranquilizers*, these medications are used to treat psychosis and severe anxiety. They also enhance the effectiveness of SSRIs. High-potency antipsychotics, can be used while feeding with breast milk. The babies should be watched for sleepiness; however, there have been no reports of infant problems. The "second generation" or atypical antipsychotics are seen in very small amounts in breast milk, and considered compatible.

Electroconvulsive Therapy (ECT)

ECT is considered an acceptable treatment for severe depression or psychosis postpartum, and does not affect breast milk. It may also be useful in treating bipolar disorder postpartum. ECT is not used for postpartum anxiety, panic, or OCD.

Mood Stabilizers

Some mood stabilizers may be safer than others while feeding with breast milk. Consult your perinatal prescriber for guidance. Children given breast milk from a mother taking an anti-epileptic medication had no adverse effects at 6 years of age (Birnbaum, 2020).

Sleep Aids

Most over-the-counter and prescribed medications used as sleep aids are found in low levels in breast milk, and are considered acceptable.

Medical Protocols

The following guidelines, based on research in the field to date, suggest treatments based on the patient's history. Treatments should be followed in sequence, with Treatment 1 tried first, followed by Treatment 2 if necessary.

Although the treatment protocols that follow refer only to depression and psychosis, they are also effective in the treatment of OCD, anxiety, and panic.

SSRIs are usually the first choice in the treatment of OCD, anxiety, and panic. It may be helpful to use low-dose antianxiety or antipsychotic medications on a short-term basis for anxiety and panic. Often high doses of SSRIs are needed, and for longer periods of time.

Refer to Chapter 7 to determine what complementary and alternative medicine (CAM) treatment(s) might be most effective for any given situation.

PRE-PREGNANCY		
History	**Treatment 1**	**Treatment 2**
One episode of major depression if on med + asymptomatic for 6–12 months	Taper off med + therapy (monitor closely for relapse) + support + CAM	Resume med + continue therapy + support + CAM
Severe recurrent prior episodes	Continue med + therapy + support + CAM	Med + therapy + support + CAM

Mild major depression or severe major depression (first episode)	Therapy + support + CAM	Therapy + med + support + CAM
Bipolar disorder	Continue or switch if on valproic acid (Depakote) or carbamazepine (Tegretol) to lithium or lamotrigine (Lamictal) + have psychiatrist monitor closely + therapy + support + CAM	Switch to high potency antipsychotic + therapy + support+ CAM

PREGNANCY (including first trimester)		
History	**Treatment 1**	**Treatment 2**
One episode of mild major depression, currently in remission	Taper off med + therapy + support + CAM	Resume med + therapy + support + CAM
One episode of severe major depression, currently in remission	Consider tapering off or maintenance of med + therapy +support + CAM	Med + therapy + support + CAM
Mild major depression, first or recurrent	Therapy + support+ CAM	Med + therapy + support + CAM
Severe major depression	Med + therapy + support + CAM	Med + therapy + support + CAM

		Consider ECT, TMS
Recurrence or relapse of mild major depression if off med	Therapy + support+ CAM	Med + therapy + support+ CAM
Psychosis in any trimester	Hospitalization + med + therapy when stable	Hospitalization Consider ECT

POSTPARTUM		
Diagnosis	**Treatment 1**	**Treatment 2**
Mild-moderate major depression/ anxiety	Therapy + support + CAM	Therapy + med+ support + CAM Consider TMS, brexanolone, zuranolone
Severe major depression/ anxiety	Therapy + SSRI + support + CAM	Consider addition of atypical antipsychotic Support + CAM, TMS, brexanolone, zuranolone
Postpartum psychosis	Hospitalization + med + therapy once stable + CAM	Hospitalization Consider medication + ECT + CAM

PREVENTION OF POSTPARTUM DEPRESSION IN WOMEN WITH HISTORY OF DEPRESSION, ANXIETY, OTHER MOOD DISORDER, OR PRIOR POSTPARTUM ILLNESS		
History	Treatment 1	Treatment 2
First pregnancy	Meet with therapist when risk identified (pre-pregnancy or pregnancy) + psychoeducation for woman and partner + CAM	Intervention (refer to pregnancy treatment protocol) if symptomatic + support + CAM
Prior postpartum depression/anxiety	Psychoeducation for woman and partner as early as possible + therapy+ support + CAM	Intervention (refer to pregnancy treatment protocol) if symptomatic + support + CAM
Prior postpartum psychosis	Refer to perinatal psychiatrist + therapy	Intervention (refer to pregnancy treatment protocol) if symptomatic

Resources

Websites and Helplines

Action on Postpartum Psychosis
app-network.org
Perinatal psychosis information and support

Childbirth and Postpartum Professional Association
CAPPA.net
Doula training and help locating a doula.

Doulas of North America
dona.org
An international, nonprofit organization of doulas that strives to have every doula trained and educated to provide the highest quality and standards for birth and/or postpartum support to birthing women and their families.

Hotline—National Maternal Mental Health Hotline
24/7, free, confidential support before, during, and after pregnancy.
Call or text 833-TLC-MAMA (833-852-6262). TTY users can use a preferred relay service or dial 711 and then 833-852-6262.)

Infant Risk HCP Mobile App (for Healthcare Providers)
infantrisk.org
Thomas Hale's website on medications in pregnancy and lactation from Texas Tech University Health Sciences Center.
MommyMeds App (Pregnancy Safety Guide) health and safety app for all pregnant and breastfeeding mothers from InfantRisk.

Marcé of North America
www.perinatalmentalhealth.com
North American branch of the International Marcé Society.

Marcé Society
marcesociety.com
The Marcé Society is an international organization dedicated to scientific research in perinatal mental health.

Massachusetts General Hospital Center for Women's Mental Health
womensmentalhealth.org
A perinatal and reproductive psychiatry information center. Massachusetts General Hospital Psychosis Project mghp3.org.

Mothertobaby.org
866-626-6847 and app
Information about medications in pregnancy and breastfeeding in English and Spanish

North American Society for Psychosocial OB/GYN
naspog.org
The North American Society for Psychosocial Obstetrics and Gynecology is a society of researchers, clinicians, educators, and scientists involved in women's mental health and healthcare.

Postpartum Dads/Partners
postpartum.net—PSI
Chat with an expert for dads and partners.

Postpartum Support International (PSI)
postpartum.net

800-944-4PPD (944-4773) #1 En Español or #2 English for voice message.

Text "Help" to 800-944-4773 (EN)

Text en Español: 971-203-7773

PSI App: Connect by PSI

Support for Prescribers Call 877-499-4773 and leave a message. Postpartum Support International is dedicated to helping parents suffering from perinatal mood and anxiety disorders, including postpartum depression, the most common complication of childbirth. PSI works to educate family, friends, and healthcare providers. *Healthy Mom, Happy Family*, a thirteen-minute educational DVD in English and Spanish, is available at postpartum.net. Many types of support groups are offered through PSI.

Shoshana Bennett's Website

DrShosh.com

Resources such as the film *Dark Side of The Full Moon* and books by Shoshana

DarkSideofTheFullMoon.com

ParentalAction.com

Parental Action Institute founded by Shoshana Bennett and Jane Honikman (Founder of PSI, janehonikman.com)

Zuranolone (Zurzuvae) Resources

Sagerx.com

Patients and prescribers can contact the Sage access line for support with Zurzuvae coverage at 844-472-4379.

Journal Articles

The articles listed in this section were written for medical professionals. They are presented here for those readers who are comfortable with medical and scientific terminology.

Abramowitz, J. A. "Obsessive-Compulsive Symptoms in Pregnancy and the Puerperium: A Review of the Literature." *Anxiety Disorders* 2003; 17:461–478.

Aldera, Hussain, et al. "Do Parental Comorbidities Affect the Severity of Autism Spectrum Disorder?" *Cureus*, vol. 14,12 e32702. 19 Dec. 2022.

Alwan S., et al. "National Birth Defects Prevention, Study. Use of Selective Serotonin-Reuptake Inhibitors in Pregnancy and the Risk of Birth Defects." *New England Journal of Medicine* 2007; 356:2684–2692.

American College of Obstetrics and Gynecology "Committee Opinion No. 722: Marijuana Use During Pregnancy and Lactation." *Obstetrics and gynecology* vol. 130,4 (2017): e205-e209.

American College of Obstetrics and Gynecology. "Use of Psychiatric Medications During Pregnancy and Lactation." *Practice Bulletin* 2008 Apr; No. 92.

Anderson, Eric L., and Irving M. Reti. "ECT in pregnancy: a review of the literature from 1941 to 2007." *Psychosomatic medicine*, vol. 71,2 (2009): 235-42.

Andrade C. "Major Congenital Malformations Associated with Exposure to Antiepilectic Drugs During Pregnancy." *The Journal of Clinical Psychiatry* 2018; 79(4):18f12449.

Andrade C. "The Safety of Duloxetine During Pregnancy and Lactation." *The Journal of Clinical Psychiatry* Dec 2014; 75(12):e1423–7.

Ansari, Najmus Sehr, et al. "Risk factors for postpartum depressive symptoms among fathers: A systematic review and meta-analysis." *Acta obstetricia et gynecologica* Scandinavica, vol. 100,7 (2021): 1186–1199.

Appleby, L., et al. "A Controlled Study of Fluoxetine and Cognitive Behavioural Counseling in the Treatment of Postnatal Depression." *British Medical Journal* 1997; 314:932–936.

Bais, Babette, et al. "Effects of bright light therapy for depression during pregnancy: a randomised, double-blind controlled trial." *BMJ open*, vol. 10,10 e038030. 28 Oct. 2020.

Bang Madson, K., et al. "In utero exposure to ADHD medication and long-term offspring outcomes." *Molecular psychiatry* 2023, *28*(4), 1739–1746.

Barrera, Alinne Z., et al. "Online prevention of postpartum depression for Spanish- and English-speaking pregnant women: A pilot randomized controlled trial." *Internet interventions*, vol. 2,3 (2015): 257–265.

Battle, C., et al. "Potential for prenatal yoga to serve as an intervention to treat depression during pregnancy." *Womens Health Issues* 2015; 25(2):134–141.

Bayrampour, Hamideh, et al. "The Risk of Relapse of Depression During Pregnancy After Discontinuation of Antidepressants: A Systematic Review and Meta-Analysis." *The Journal of clinical psychiatry* vol. 81,4 19r13134. 9 Jun. 2020.

Beck, C. T. "Impact of Birth Trauma on Breastfeeding." *Nursing Research* 2008; 57(4):228–236.

Beck, C. T., and R. Gable. "Postpartum Depression Screening Scale (PDSS)." Available through Western Psychological Services, 800-648–8857.

Beck, Cheryl Tatano, and Pec Indman. "The many faces of postpartum depression." *Journal of obstetric, gynecologic, and neonatal nursing: JOGNN*, vol. 34,5 (2005): 569–76.

Beck, Cheryl Tatano, et al. "Traumatic Childbirth and Its Aftermath: Is There Anything Positive?" *The Journal of perinatal education*, vol. 27,3 (2018): 175–184.

Bennett, H. A. "Prevalence of Depression During Pregnancy. Systematic Review." *American College of Obstetricians and Gynecologists* Apr 2004; 103:698–709.

Bennett H. A., et al. "Prevalence of Depression During Pregnancy. Overview of Clinical Factors." *Clinical Drug Investigations* 2004; 24 (3): 157–179.

Bennett, Shoshana, et al. "Use of modified spectacles and light bulbs to block blue light at night may prevent postpartum depression." *Medical hypotheses*, vol. 73,2 (2009): 251–3.

Benyshek, Daniel C., et al. "Comparison of placenta consumers' and non-consumers' postpartum depression screening results using EPDS in US community birth settings (n=6038): a propensity score analysis." *BMC pregnancy and childbirth*, vol. 23,1 534. 22 Jul. 2023.

Bergink, V., et al. "Prevention of Postpartum Psychosis and Mania in Women at High Risk." *American Journal of Psychiatry* 2012; 169:609–15.

Berle, J. O., et al. "Neonatal Outcomes in Offspring of Women with Anxiety and Depression During Pregnancy." *Archives of Women's Mental Health* 2005; 8:181–189.

Besag, Frank M. C., and Michael J. Vasey. "Should Antidepressants be Avoided in Pregnancy?" *Drug safety*, vol. 46,1 (2023): 1–17.

Birnbaum, Angela K., et al. "Antiepileptic Drug Exposure in Infants of Breastfeeding Mothers With Epilepsy." *JAMA neurology*, vol. 77,4 (2020): 441–450.

Bodnar, L., and Katherine Wisner. "Nutrition and Depression: Implications for Improving Mental Health Among Childbearing-Aged Women." *Biological Psychiatry* 2005; 58:679–685.

Borja-Hart, N. L., and Jehan Marino. "Role of Omega-3 Fatty Acids for Prevention or Treatment of Perinatal Depression." *Pharmacotherapy* 2010; 30(2):210–216.

Borri, C., et al. "Axis I Psychopathology and Functional Impairment at the Third Month of Pregnancy: Results from the Perinatal Depression-Research and Screening Unit (PND-ReScU) Study." *The Journal of Clinical Psychiatry* 2008; 69:1617–1624.

Boyd, R. C., et al. "Review of screening instruments for postpartum depression." *Archives of women's mental health*, vol. 8,3 (2005): 141–53.

Boyle, Breidge, et al. "The changing epidemiology of Ebstein's anomaly and its relationship with maternal mental health conditions: a European registry-based study." *Cardiology in the young*, vol. 27,4 (2017): 677–685.

Brandon, A. R., et al. "Nonpharmacologic Treatments for Depression Related to Reproductive Events." *Current Psychiatry Reports* Oct 2014; 16:526.

Brennan, Patricia A., et al. "Prenatal Antidepressant Exposures and Autism Spectrum Disorder or Traits: A Retrospective, Multi-Cohort Study." *Research on child and adolescent psychopathology*, vol. 51,4 (2023); 513–527.

Bright, Katherine S., et al. "Interpersonal Psychotherapy to Reduce Psychological Distress in Perinatal Women: A Systematic Review." *International journal of environmental research and public health*, vol. 17,22 8421. 13 Nov. 2020.

Brockington, Ian. "Suicide and filicide in postpartum psychosis." *Archives of Women's Mental Health* 2017; 20:63–69.

Byatt N., et al. "Antidepressant Use in Pregnancy: A Critical Review Focused on Risks and Controversies." *Acta Psychiatrica Scandinavica* 2013; 127:94–114.

CDC. https://www.cdc.gov/reproductivehealth/maternal-mortality/erase-mm/data-mmrc.html.

Chan, Adrienne Y. L., et al. "Maternal Benzodiazepines and Z-Drugs Use during Pregnancy and Adverse Birth and Neurodevelopmental Outcomes in Offspring: A Population-Based Cohort Study." *Psychotherapy and psychosomatics*, vol. 92,2 (2023): 113–123.

Chaudron, Linda H, and Neha Nirodi. "The obsessive-compulsive spectrum in the perinatal period: a prospective pilot study." *Archives of women's mental health*, vol. 13,5 (2010): 403–10.

Chen, Qianqian, et al. "Prevalence and Risk Factors Associated with Postpartum Depression during the COVID-19 Pandemic: A Literature Review and Meta-Analysis." *International journal of environmental research and public health*, vol. 19,4 2219. 16 Feb. 2022.

Chin, Kathleen, et al. "Suicide and Maternal Mortality." *Current psychiatry reports*, vol. 24,4 (2022); 239–275.

Chiu, Chih-Chiang, et al. "Omega-3 fatty acids for depression in pregnancy." *The American journal of psychiatry*, vol. 160,2 (2003): 385.

Cohen, L. S., et al. "Relapse of depression during pregnancy following antidepressant discontinuation: a preliminary prospective study." *Archives of women's mental health*, vol. 7,4 (2004): 217–21.

Cohen, L. S., et al. "Venlafaxine in the treatment of postpartum depression." *The Journal of clinical psychiatry*, vol. 62,8 (2001): 592–6.

Cohen, Lee S., et al. "Relapse of major depression during pregnancy in women who maintain or discontinue antidepressant treatment." *JAMA*, vol. 295,5 (2006).

Corral, M., et al. "Morning light therapy for postpartum depression." *Archives of women's mental health*, vol. 10,5 (2007): 221–4.

Cox, J. L., et al. "Detection of postnatal depression. Development of the 10-item Edinburgh Postnatal Depression Scale." *The British journal of psychiatry: the journal of mental science*, vol. 150 (1987): 782–6.

Croen, Lisa A., et al. "Antidepressant use during pregnancy and childhood autism spectrum disorders." *Archives of general psychiatry*, vol. 68,11 (2011): 1104–12.

Dagher, Rada K., et al. "Perinatal Depression: Challenges and Opportunities." *Journal of women's health (2002)*, vol. 30,2 (2021): 154–159.

Damkier, Per, and Poul Videbech. "The Safety of Second-Generation Antipsychotics During Pregnancy: A Clinically Focused Review." *CNS drugs*, vol. 32,4 (2018): 351–366.

Dehkordi, Z. R. "The Effects of Infant Massage on Maternal Postpartum Depression: A Randomized Controlled Trial." *Nursing and Midwifery Studies* 2019; 8(1):28–33.

Deligiannidis, Kristina M, and Marlene P Freeman. "Complementary and alternative medicine therapies for perinatal depression." *Best practice & research. Clinical obstetrics & gynaecology*, vol. 28,1 (2014): 85–95.

Deligiannidis, Kristina M., et al. "Zuranolone for the Treatment of Postpartum Depression." *The American journal of psychiatry*, vol. 180,9 (2023): 668–675.

Dennis, Cindy-Lee, and Therese Dowswell. "Psychosocial and psychological interventions for preventing postpartum depression." *The Cochrane database of systematic reviews*, 2 CD001134. 28 Feb. 2013.

DeRosa, Nancy, and M. Cynthia Logsdon. "A comparison of screening instruments for depression in postpartum adolescents." *Journal of child and adolescent psychiatric nursing: official publication of the Association of Child and Adolescent Psychiatric Nurses, Inci,* vol. 19,1 (2006): 13–20.

Doan, Therese, et al. "Breast-feeding increases sleep duration of new parents." *The Journal of perinatal & neonatal nursing,* vol. 21,3 (2007): 200–6.

Donmez, Melike, et al. "Efficacy of bright light therapy in perinatal depression: A randomized, double-blind, placebo-controlled study." *Journal of psychiatric research,* vol. 149 (2022): 315–322.

Earls, M. F., et al. "Incorporating Recognition and Management of Perinatal Depression Into Pediatric Practice." https://pediatrics.aappublications.org/content/pediatrics/143/1/e20183259.full.pdf.

Einarson, A. "Antipsychotic Medication (Safety/Risk) During Pregnancy and Breastfeeding." *Current Women's Health Reviews,* vol. 6 (1) (2010).

Einarson, Adrienne. "Paroxetine use in pregnancy and increased risk of heart defects: Evaluating the evidence." *Canadian family physician Medecin de famille canadien*, vol. 56,8 (2010): 767–8.

Einarson, Adrienne, et al. "Incidence of major malformations in infants following antidepressant exposure in pregnancy: results of a large prospective cohort study." *Canadian journal of psychiatry. Revue canadienne de psychiatrie*, vol. 54,4 (2009): 242–6.

Eleftheriou, Georgios, et al. "Consensus Panel Recommendations for the Pharmacological Management of Pregnant Women with Depressive Disorders." *International journal of environmental research and public health*, vol. 20,16 6565. 11 Aug. 2023.

Ersek, Jennifer L, and Larissa R Brunner Huber. "Physical activity prior to and during pregnancy and risk of postpartum depressive symptoms." *Journal of obstetric, gynecologic, and neonatal nursing: JOGNN*, vol. 38,5 (2009): 556–66.

Esaki, Yuichi, et al. "A double-blind, randomized, placebo-controlled trial of adjunctive blue-blocking glasses for the treatment of sleep and circadian rhythm in patients with bipolar disorder." *Bipolar disorders*, vol. 22,7 (2020): 739–748.

Fairbrother, Nichole, et al. "Perinatal anxiety disorder prevalence and incidence." *Journal of affective disorders*, vol. 200 (2016): 148–55.

Falconi, April M., et al. "Doula care across the maternity care continuum and impact on maternal health: Evaluation of doula programs across three states using propensity score matching." *EClinicalMedicine*, vol. 50 101531. 1 Jul. 2022.

Fang, Qian, et al. "Effect of peer support intervention on perinatal depression: A meta-analysis." *General hospital psychiatry*, vol. 74 (2022): 78–87.

Felder, Jennifer N., et al. "Efficacy of Digital Cognitive Behavioral Therapy for the Treatment of Insomnia Symptoms Among Pregnant Women: A Randomized Clinical Trial." *JAMA psychiatry*, vol. 77,5 (2020): 484–492.

Felder, Jennifer N. et al. "Endorsement of a single-item measure of sleep disturbance during pregnancy and risk for postpartum depression: a retrospective cohort study." *Archives of women's mental health*, vol. 26,1 (2023): 67–74.

Field, T. "Maternal depression effects on infants and early interventions." *Preventive medicine*, vol. 27,2 (1998): 200–3.

Field, Tiffany. "Postpartum depression effects on early interactions, parenting, and safety practices: a review." *Infant behavior & development*, vol. 33,1 (2010): 1–6.

Field, Tiffany, et al. "Chronic prenatal depression and neonatal outcome." *The International journal of neuroscience*, vol. 118,1 (2008): 95–103.

Field, Tiffany, et al. "Prenatal dysthymia versus major depression effects on the neonate." *Infant behavior & development*, vol. 31,2 (2008): 190–3.

Fisher, Sheehan D. "Paternal Mental Health: Why Is It Relevant?" *American journal of lifestyle* medicine, vol. 11,3 200-211. 16 Feb. 2016.

Forman, David R., et al. "Effective treatment for postpartum depression is not sufficient to improve the developing mother-child relationship." *Development and psychopathology*, vol. 19,2 (2007): 585602.

Freeman, Marlene P. "Breastfeeding and antidepressants: clinical dilemmas and expert perspectives." *The Journal of clinical psychiatry*, vol. 70,2 (2009): 291–2.

Freeman, Marlene P. "Omega-3 fatty acids: an ideal treatment for depression in pregnancy?" *Evidence-Based Integrative Medicine* 1 (2004): 43–49.

Freeman, Marlene P., et al. "A prenatal supplement with methylfolate for the treatment and prevention of depression in women trying to conceive and during pregnancy." *Annals of clinical psychiatry, official journal of the American Academy of Clinical Psychiatrists*, vol. 31,1 (2019): 4–16.

Freeman, Marlene P., et al. "Omega-3 fatty acids and supportive psychotherapy for perinatal depression: a randomized placebo-controlled study." *Journal of affective disorders*, vol. 110,1–2 (2008): 142–8.

Friedrich, Joseph, et al. "The grass isn't always greener: The effects of cannabis on embryological development." *BMC pharmacology & toxicology*, vol. 17,1 45. 29 Sep. 2016.

Gao, Shan-Yan, et al. "Selective serotonin reuptake inhibitor use during early pregnancy and congenital malformations: a systematic review and meta-analysis of cohort studies of more than 9 million births." *BMC medicine*, vol. 16,1 205. 12 Nov. 2018.

Garbazza, Corrado., et al. "Sustained remission from perinatal depression after bright light therapy: A pilot randomised, placebo-controlled trial." *Acta psychiatrica Scandinavica*, vol. 146,4 (2022): 350–356.

Gavin, Norma I., et al. "Perinatal depression: a systematic review of prevalence and incidence." *Obstetrics and gynecology*, vol. 106,5 Pt 1 (2005): 1071–83.

Geary, Orla, et al. "The effectiveness of mother-led infant massage on symptoms of maternal postnatal depression: A systematic review." *PloS one*, vol. 18,12 e0294156. 13 Dec. 2023.

Gjerdingen, Dwenda K, and Barbara P Yawn. "Postpartum depression screening: importance, methods, barriers, and recommendations for practice." *Journal of the American Board of Family Medicine: JABFM*, vol. 20,3 (2007): 280–8.

Gjerdingen, Dwenda, et al. "Postpartum depression screening at well-child visits: validity of a 2-question screen and the PHQ-9." *Annals of family medicine*, vol. 7,1 (2009): 63–70.

Glover, Vivette, and Thomas G O'Connor. "Effects of antenatal stress and anxiety: Implications for development and psychiatry." *The British journal of psychiatry: the journal of mental science*, vol. 180 (2002): 389–91.

Grigoriadis, S., et al. "Benzodiazepine Use During Pregnancy Alone or in Combination With an Antidepressant and Congenital Malformations: Systematic Review and Meta-Analysis." *The Journal of clinical psychiatry*, vol. 80,4 18r12412. 9 Jul. 2019.

Grigoriadis, Sophie, et al. "Antidepressant exposure during pregnancy and congenital malformations: is there an association? A systematic review and meta-analysis of the best evidence." *The Journal of clinical psychiatry*, vol. 74,4 (2013): e293–308.

Grigoriadis, Sophie et al. "The effect of prenatal antidepressant exposure on neonatal adaptation: a systematic review and meta-analysis." *The Journal of clinical psychiatry*, vol. 74,4 (2013): e309–20.

Grigoriadis, Sophie et al. "The impact of maternal depression during pregnancy on perinatal outcomes: a systematic review and meta-analysis." *The Journal of clinical psychiatry*, vol. 74,4 (2013): e321–41.

Grzeskowiak, L. E., et al. "Continuation versus Cessation of Antidepressant Use in the Pre- and Post-Natal Period and Impact on Duration of Breastfeeding. Birth Defects Research Part A." *Clinical and Molecular Teratology* 2014; 100:538–539.

Gunlicks, Meredith L, and Myrna M Weissman. "Change in child psychopathology with improvement in parental depression: a systematic review." *Journal of the American Academy of Child and Adolescent Psychiatry*, vol. 47,4 (2008): 379–389.

Gunn, J. K. L., et al. "Prenatal exposure to cannabis and maternal and child health outcomes: a systematic review and meta-analysis." *BMJ open*, vol. 6,4 e009986. 5 Apr. 2016.

Gutierrez-Galve, Leticia et al. "Association of Maternal and Paternal Depression in the Postnatal Period With Offspring Depression at Age 18 Years." *JAMA psychiatry*, vol. 76,3 (2019): 290–296.

Halushka, P. "St. John's Wort: A Mini-Review of Its Pharmocokinetics and Anti-Depressant Effects. https://www.medscape.com/viewarticle/713605.

Hammen, Constance, and Patricia A Brennan. "Severity, chronicity, and timing of maternal depression and risk for adolescent offspring diagnoses in a community sample." *Archives of general psychiatry*, vol. 60,3 (2003): 253–8.

Hantsoo, Liisa, et al. "A randomized, placebo-controlled, double-blind trial of sertraline for postpartum depression." *Psychopharmacology*, vol. 231,5 (2014): 93948.

Hay, Dale F., et al. "Mothers' antenatal depression and their children's antisocial outcomes." *Child development,* vol. 81,1 (2010): 149–65.

Hendrick, Victoria, and Lori Altshuler. "Management of major depression during pregnancy." *The American journal of psychiatry,* vol. 159,10 (2002): 1667–73.

Hodgkinson, Stacy C., et al. "Depressive symptoms and birth outcomes among pregnant teenagers." *Journal of pediatric and adolescent gynecology,* vol. 23,1 (2010): 16–22.

Hudepohl, Neha, et al. "Perinatal Obsessive-Compulsive Disorder: Epidemiology, Phenomenology, Etiology, and Treatment." *Current psychiatry reports,* vol. 24,4 (2022): 229–237.

Huybrechts, Krista F., et al. "Association Between Methylphenidate and Amphetamine Use in Pregnancy and Risk of Congenital Malformations: A Cohort Study From the International Pregnancy Safety Study Consortium." *JAMA psychiatry,* vol. 75,2 (2018): 167–175.

Huybrechts, Krista F., et al. "Association of In Utero Antipsychotic Medication Exposure With Risk of Congenital Malformations in Nordic Countries and the US." *JAMA psychiatry,* vol. 80,2 (2023): 156–166.

Hviid, Anders et al. "Use of selective serotonin reuptake inhibitors during pregnancy and risk of autism." *The New England journal of medicine,* vol. 369,25 (2013): 2406–15.

Janecka, Magdalena, et al. "Association of Autism Spectrum Disorder With Prenatal Exposure to Medication Affecting Neurotransmitter Systems." *JAMA psychiatry,* vol. 75,12 (2018): 1217–1224.

Jaques, S. C., et al. "Cannabis, the pregnant woman and her child: weeding out the myths." *Journal of perinatology: official journal of the California Perinatal Association*, vol. 34,6 (2014): 417–24.

Kendig, S., et al. "Consensus Bundle on Maternal Mental Health: Perinatal Depression and Anxiety." *Journal of The American College of Obstetricians and Gynecologists* 2017; 0:1–9.

Koren, Gideon, and Hedvig Nordeng. "Antidepressant use during pregnancy: the benefit-risk ratio." *American journal of obstetrics and gynecology*, vol. 207,3 (2012): 157–63.

Koren, Gideon et al. "Is maternal use of selective serotonin reuptake inhibitors in the third trimester of pregnancy harmful to neonates?" *CMAJ: Canadian Medical Association journal = journal de l'Association medicale Canadienne*, vol. 172,11 (2005): 1457–9.

Kronenfeld, Nirit, et al. "Chronic use of psychotropic medications in breastfeeding women: Is it safe?" *PloS one*, vol. 13,5 e0197196. 21 May. 2018.

Lanza di Scalea, Teresa, and Katherine L Wisner. "Antidepressant medication use during breastfeeding." *Clinical obstetrics and* gynecology, vol. 52,3 (2009): 483–97.

Larsen, Søren Vinther, et al. "Depression Associated With Hormonal Contraceptive Use as a Risk Indicator for Postpartum Depression." *JAMA psychiatry*, vol. 80,7 (2023): 682–689.

Leng, Ling Li., et al. "Antenatal mobile-delivered mindfulness-based intervention to reduce perinatal depression risk and improve obstetric and neonatal outcomes: A randomized controlled trial." *Journal of affective disorders*, vol. 335 (2023): 216–227.

Lewandowski, R. Eric, et al. "Predictors of Positive Outcomes in Offspring of Depressed Parents and Non-depressed Parents

Across 20 Years." *Journal of child and family studies,* vol. 23,5 (2014): 800–811.

Li, Wei, et al. "Effectiveness of Acupuncture Used for the Management of Postpartum Depression: A Systematic Review and Meta-Analysis." *BioMed research international,* vol. 2019 6597503. 20 Mar. 2019.

Li, Xinyuan, et al. "Effectiveness of cognitive behavioral therapy for perinatal maternal depression, anxiety and stress: A systematic review and meta-analysis of randomized controlled trials." *Clinical psychology review,* vol. 92 (2022): 102129.

Lindahl, V., et al. "Prevalence of suicidality during pregnancy and the postpartum." *Archives of women's mental healthi,* vol. 8,2 (2005): 77–87.

Louik, Carol, et al. "First-trimester use of selective serotonin-reuptake inhibitors and the risk of birth defects." *The New England journal of medicine,* vol. 356,26 (2007): 2675–83.

Manber, Rachel, et al. "Acupuncture for depression during pregnancy: a randomized controlled trial." *Obstetrics and gynecology,* vol. 115,3 (2010): 511–520.

Marchand, Greg, et al. "Birth Outcomes of Neonates Exposed to Marijuana in Utero: A Systematic Review and Meta-analysis." *JAMA network open,* vol. 5,1 e2145653. 4 Jan. 2022.

Marcus, Sheila M. "Depression during pregnancy: rates, risks and consequences—Motherisk Update 2008." *The Canadian journal of clinical pharmacology,* vol. 16,1 (2009): e15–22.

Marcus, Sheila M., et al. "Depressive symptoms among pregnant women screened in obstetrics settings." *Journal of women's health (2002),* vol. 12,4 (2003): 373–80.

Maschi, S., et al. "Neonatal outcome following pregnancy exposure to antidepressants: a prospective controlled cohort study." *BJOG: an international journal of obstetrics and gynaecology*, vol. 115,2 (2008): 28–39.

Maxfield, Louise. "A Clinician's Guide to the Efficacy of EMDR Therapy." *Journal of EMDR Practice and Research* 13 (2019): 239–246.

McKenna, Kate, et al. "Pregnancy outcome of women using atypical antipsychotic drugs: a prospective comparative study." *The Journal of clinical psychiatry*, vol. 66,4 (2005): 444–9.

Meador, Kimford J., et al. "Cognitive function at 3 years of age after fetal exposure to antiepileptic drugs." *The New England journal of medicine*, vol. 360,16 (2009): 1597–605.

Meltzer-Brody, Samantha, and Alison Stuebe. "The long-term psychiatric and medical prognosis of perinatal mental illness." *Best practice & research. Clinical obstetrics & gynaecology*, vol. 28,1 (2014): 49–60.

Meng, Lin-Chieh et al. "Benzodiazepine Use During Pregnancy and Risk of Miscarriage." *JAMA psychiatry* vol. 81,4 (2024): 366-373.

Metz, Torri D., et al. "Cannabis Exposure and Adverse Pregnancy Outcomes Related to Placental Function." *JAMA*, vol. 330,22 (2023): 2191–2199.

Michalczyk, Justyna, et al. "Postpartum Psychosis: A Review of Risk Factors, Clinical Picture, Management, Prevention, and Psychosocial Determinants." *Medical science monitor: international medical journal of experimental and clinical research*, vol. 29 e942520. 29 Dec. 2023.

Mitchell, J. and J. Goodman. "Comparative effects of antidepressant medications and untreated major depression on pregnancy outcomes: a systematic review." *Archives of Women's Mental Health* Apr 2018; 21(5); 505–516.

Miuli, Andrea, et al. "Beyond the efficacy of transcranial magnetic stimulation in peripartum depression: A systematic review exploring perinatal safety for newborns." *Psychiatry research*, vol. 326 (2023): 115251.

Momen, Natalie C., et al. "In utero exposure to antipsychotic medication and psychiatric outcomes in the offspring." *Neuropsychopharmacology: official publication of the American College of Neuropsychopharmacology*, vol. 47,3 (2022): 759–766.

Moretti, Myla E., et al. "Evaluating the safety of St. John's Wort in human pregnancy." *Reproductive toxicology (Elmsford, N.Y.)*, vol. 28,1 (2009): 96–9.

Morris, Emily, et al. "A Matched Cohort Study of Postpartum Placentophagy in Women With a History of Mood Disorders: No Evidence for Impact on Mood, Energy, Vitamin B_{12} Levels, or Lactation." *Journal of obstetrics and gynaecology Canada: JOGC = Journal d'obstetrique et gynecologie du Canada: JOGC*, vol. 41,9 (2019): 1330–1337.

Moses-Kolko, Eydie L., et al. "Neonatal signs after late in utero exposure to serotonin reuptake inhibitors: literature review and implications for clinical applications." *JAMA*, vol. 293,19 (2005): 2372–83.

Moses-Kolko, Eydie L., et al. "Transdermal estradiol for postpartum depression: a promising treatment option." *Clinical obstetrics and gynecology*, vol. 52,3 (2009): 516–29.

Moss, Michael J., et al. "Cannabis use and measurement of cannabinoids in plasma and breast milk of breastfeeding mothers." *Pediatric research*, vol. 90,4 (2021): 861–868.

Mounts, Kyle O. "Screening for maternal depression in the neonatal ICU." *Clinics in perinatology*, vol. 36,1 (2009): 137–52.

Mulcahy, Rhiannon, et al. "A randomised control trial for the effectiveness of group Interpersonal Psychotherapy for postnatal depression." *Archives of women's mental health*, vol. 13,2 (2010): 125–39.

Netsi, Elena, et al. "Association of Persistent and Severe Postnatal Depression With Child Outcomes." *JAMA psychiatry*, vol. 75,3 (2018): 247–253.

Newport, D. Jeffrey, et al. "Lamotrigine in breast milk and nursing infants: determination of exposure." *Pediatrics*, vol. 122,1 (2008): e223–31.

Nordeng, Hedvig, and Olav Spigset. "Treatment with Selective Serotonin Reuptake Inhibitors in the Third Trimester of Pregnancy: Effects on the Infant." *Drug safety*, vol. 28,7 (2005): 565–581.

Norhayati, M. N., et al. "Magnitude and risk factors for postpartum symptoms: a literature review." *Journal of affective disorders*, vol. 175 (2015): 34–52.

Norman, Emily, et al. "An exercise and education program improves well-being of new mothers: a randomized controlled trial." *Physical therapy*, vol. 90,3 (2010): 348–55.

Nulman, Irena, et al. "Child development following exposure to tricyclic antidepressants or fluoxetine throughout fetal life: a prospective, controlled study." *The American journal of psychiatry*, vol. 159,11 (2002): 1889–95.

Nulman, Irena et al. "Neurodevelopment of children following prenatal exposure to venlafaxine, selective serotonin reuptake inhibitors, or untreated maternal depression." *The American journal of psychiatry*, vol. 169,11 (2012): 1165–74.

Oates, Margaret. "Perinatal psychiatric disorders: a leading cause of maternal morbidity and mortality." *British medical bulletin*, vol. 67 (2003): 219–29.

Occhiogrosso, Mallay, et al. "Persistent pulmonary hypertension of the newborn and selective serotonin reuptake inhibitors: lessons from clinical and translational studies." *The American journal of psychiatry*, vol. 169,2 (2012): 134–40.

O'Hara, M. W., et al. "Efficacy of interpersonal psychotherapy for postpartum depression." *Archives of general psychiatry*, vol. 57,11 (2000): 1039–45.

Oren, Dan A., et al. "An open trial of morning light therapy for treatment of antepartum depression." *The American journal of psychiatry*, vol. 159,4 (2002): 666–9.

Ormsby, Simone M., et al. "The feasibility of acupuncture as an adjunct intervention for antenatal depression: a pragmatic randomised controlled trial." *Journal of affective disorders*, vol. 275 (2020): 82–93.

Ornoy, Asher, and Gideon Koren. "Selective Serotonin Reuptake Inhibitors during Pregnancy: Do We Have Now More Definite Answers Related to Prenatal Exposure?." *Birth defects research*, vol. 109,12 (2017): 898–908.

Orr, Suezanne T., et al. "Maternal prenatal depressive symptoms and spontaneous preterm births among African-American women in Baltimore, Maryland." *American journal of epidemiology*, vol. 156,9 (2002): 797–802.

Orsolini, Laura, et al. "Suicide during Perinatal Period: Epidemiology, Risk Factors, and Clinical Correlates." *Frontiers in psychiatry*, vol. 7 138. 12 Aug. 2016.

Palladino, Christie Lancaster, et al. "Homicide and suicide during the perinatal period: findings from the National Violent

Death Reporting System." *Obstetrics and gynecology*, vol. 118,5 (2011): 1056–1063.

Paulson, James F., et al. "Individual and combined effects of postpartum depression in mothers and fathers on parenting behavior." *Pediatrics*, vol. 118,2 (2006): 659–68.

Pedersen, L. H., et al. "Prenatal antidepressant exposure and behavioral problems in early childhood--a cohort study." *Acta psychiatrica Scandinavica*, vol. 127,2 (2013): 126–35.

Philpott, Lloyd Frank, et al. "Anxiety in fathers in the perinatal period: A systematic review." Midwifery, vol. 76 (2019): 54–101.

Pinheiro, Emily, et al. "Sertraline and breastfeeding: review and meta-analysis." *Archives of women's mental health*, vol. 18,2 (2015): 139–146.

Pope, Carley J, and Dwight Mazmanian. "Breastfeeding and Postpartum Depression: An Overview and Methodological Recommendations for Future Research." *Depression research and treatment*, vol. 2016 (2016): 4765310.

Pope, Carley J., et al. "Recognition, diagnosis and treatment of postpartum bipolar depression." *Expert review of neurotherapeutics*, vol. 14,1 (2014): 19–28.

Prom, Maria C., et al. "A Systematic Review of Interventions That Integrate Perinatal Mental Health Care Into Routine Maternal Care in Low- and Middle-Income Countries." *Frontiers in psychiatry*, vol. 13 859341, 14 Mar. 2022.

Qiao, Y., et al. "Effects of depressive and anxiety symptoms during pregnancy on pregnant, obstetric and neonatal outcomes: a follow-up study." *Journal of obstetrics and gynaecology: the journal of the Institute of Obstetrics and Gynaecology*, vol. 32,3 (2012): 237–40.

Ramchandani, Paul G., et al. "Depression in men in the postnatal period and later child psychopathology: a population cohort study." *Journal of the American Academy of Child and Adolescent Psychiatry*, vol. 47,4 (2008): 390–398.

Reck, C., et al. "Prevalence, onset and comorbidity of postpartum anxiety and depressive disorders." *Acta psychiatrica Scandinavica*, vol. 118,6 (2008): 459–68.

Robinson, Gail Erlick. "Controversies about the use of antidepressants in pregnancy." *Journal of nervous and mental disease*, vol. 203,3 (2015): 159–63.

Ronen, Keshet, et al. "Acceptability and Utility of a Digital Group Intervention to Prevent Perinatal Depression in Youths via Interactive Maternal Group for Information and Emotional Support (IMAGINE): Pilot Cohort Study." *JMIR formative research*, vol. 8 e51066. 2 Feb. 2024.

Rose, Sherrill, et al. "Electroconvulsive Therapy in Pregnancy: Safety, Best Practices, and Barriers to Care." *Obstetrical & gynecological survey*, vol. 75,3 (2020): 199–203.

Ross, Lori E., et al. "Selected pregnancy and delivery outcomes after exposure to antidepressant medication: a systematic review and meta-analysis." *JAMA psychiatry*, vol. 70,4 (2013): 436-43.

Ross, Lori E., et al. "Sleep and perinatal mood disorders: a critical review." *Journal of psychiatry & neuroscience: JPN*, vol. 30,4 (2005): 247–56.

Rubin-Miller, Lily, et al. "Utilization of digital prenatal services and management of depression and anxiety during pregnancy: A retrospective observational study." *Frontiers in digital health*, vol. 5 1152525, 30 Mar. 2023.

Russell, Emily J., et al. "Risk of obsessive-compulsive disorder in pregnant and postpartum women: a meta-analysis." *The Journal of clinical psychiatry*, vol. 74,4 (2013): 377–85.

Ryan, Sheryl A., et al. "Marijuana Use During Pregnancy and Breastfeeding: Implications for Neonatal and Childhood Outcomes." *Pediatrics*, vol. 142,3 (2018): e20181889.

Sanz, Emilio J., et al. "Selective serotonin reuptake inhibitors in pregnant women and neonatal withdrawal syndrome: a database analysis." *Lancet (London, England)*, vol. 365,9458 (2005): 482–7.

Sarris, Jerome, and Marlene P Freeman. "Omega-3 Fatty Acid Supplementation for Perinatal Depression and Other Subpopulations?" *The Journal of clinical psychiatry*, vol. 81,5 20com13489. 1 Sep. 2020.

Segre, L. S., et al. "Interpersonal Psychotherapy for Antenatal and Postpartum Depression." *Primary Psychiatry* 2004; 11(3):52–56.

Sharma, Verinder, et al. "Bipolar II postpartum depression: Detection, diagnosis, and treatment." *The American journal of psychiatry*, vol. 166,11 (2009): 1217–21.

Shaw, Richard J., et al. "The relationship between acute stress disorder and posttraumatic stress disorder in the neonatal intensive care unit." *Psychosomatics*, vol. 50,2 (2009): 131–7.

Sheng, Zhihao, et al. "Potential CSF biomarkers of postpartum depression following delivery via caesarian section." *Journal of affective* disorders, vol. 342 (2023): 177–181.

Shi, Peixia, et al. "Maternal depression and suicide at immediate prenatal and early postpartum periods and psychosocial risk factors." *Psychiatry research* vol. 261 (2018): 298–306.

Shi, Yuyan, et al. "The associations between prenatal cannabis use disorder and neonatal outcomes." *Addiction (Abingdon, England)*, vol. 116,11 (2021): 3069–3079.

Schiller, Crystal Edler, et al. "The role of reproductive hormones in postpartum depression." *CNS spectrums*, vol. 20,1 (2015): 48–59.

Sidebottom, Abbey C., et al. "Validation of the Patient Health Questionnaire (PHQ)-9 for prenatal depression screening." *Archives of women's mental health*, vol. 15,5 (2012): 367–74.

Sit, Dorothy K Y, and Katherine L Wisner. "Identification of postpartum depression." *Clinical obstetrics and gynecology*, vol. 52,3 (2009): 456–68.

Smit, Mirte, et al. "Mirtazapine in pregnancy and lactation: data from a case series." *Journal of clinical psychopharmacology*, vol. 35,2 (2015): 163–7.

Smith, Sophie, et al. "Association between antidepressant use during pregnancy and miscarriage: a systematic review and meta-analysis." *BMJ open*, vol. 14,1 e074600. 25 Jan. 2024.

Sockol, Laura E. "A systematic review and meta-analysis of interpersonal psychotherapy for perinatal women." *Journal of affective disorders*, vol. 232 (2018): 316–328.

Sørensen, Merete Juul, et al. "Antidepressant exposure in pregnancy and risk of autism spectrum disorders." *Clinical epidemiology*, vol. 5 449-59. 15 Nov. 2013.

Sorkhou, Maryam, et al. "Birth, cognitive and behavioral effects of intrauterine cannabis exposure in infants and children: A systematic review and meta-analysis." *Addiction (Abingdon, England)*, 10.1111/add.16370. 15 Nov. 2023.

Spinelli, Margaret G., and Jean Endicott. "Controlled clinical trial of interpersonal psychotherapy versus parenting education program for depressed pregnant women." *The American journal of psychiatry*, vol. 160,3 (2003): 555–62.

Sprague, Jennifer, et al. "Pharmacotherapy for depression and bipolar disorder during lactation: A framework to aid decision making." *Seminars in perinatology*, vol. 44,3 (2020): 151224.

Stamou, George, et al. "Cognitive-Behavioural therapy and interpersonal psychotherapy for the treatment of post-natal depression: a narrative review." *BMC psychology*, vol. 6,1 28. 18 Jun. 2018.

Stevens, Anja W. M. M., et al. "Risk of recurrence of mood disorders during pregnancy and the impact of medication: A systematic review." *Journal of affective disorders*, vol. 249 (2019): 96–103.

Straub, Loreen, et al., "Association of Antipsychotic Drug Exposure in Pregnancy With Risk of Neurodevelopmental Disorders: A National Birth Cohort Study." *JAMA internal medicine*, vol. 182,5 (2022): 522–533.

Stuart, S., et al. "The prevention and psychotherapeutic treatment of postpartum depression." *Archives of women's mental health*, vol. 6 Suppl 2 (2003): S57–69.

Sundbakk, Lene Maria, et al. "Association of Prenatal Exposure to Benzodiazepines and Z-Hypnotics With Risk of Attention-Deficit/Hyperactivity Disorder in Childhood." *JAMA network open*, vol. 5,12 e2246889. 1 Dec. 2022.

Suri, Rita, et al. "Effects of antenatal depression and antidepressant treatment on gestational age at birth and risk of preterm birth." *The American journal of psychiatry*, vol. 164,8 (2007): 1206–13.

Szpunar, Mercedes J., et al. "Risk of major malformations in infants after first-trimester exposure to benzodiazepines: Results from the Massachusetts General Hospital National Pregnancy Registry for Psychiatric Medications." *Depression and anxiety*, vol. 39,12 (2022).

Tak, Casey R., et al. "The impact of exposure to antidepressant medications during pregnancy on neonatal outcomes: a review of retrospective database cohort studies." *European journal of clinical pharmacology*, vol. 73,9 (2017): 1055–1069.

Van den Bergh, Bea R. H., et al. "Antenatal maternal anxiety and stress and the neurobehavioural development of the fetus and child: links and possible mechanisms. A review." *Neuroscience and biobehavioral reviews*, vol. 29,2 (2005): 237–58.

Van Lieshout, Ryan J., et al. "Effect of Online 1-Day Cognitive Behavioral Therapy-Based Workshops Plus Usual Care vs Usual Care Alone for Postpartum Depression: A Randomized Clinical Trial." *JAMA psychiatry*, vol. 78,11 (2021): 1200–1207.

Viguera, Adele C., et al. "Risk of recurrence in women with bipolar disorder during pregnancy: prospective study of mood stabilizer discontinuation." *The American journal of psychiatry*, vol. 164,12 (2007): 1817–24.

Villar-Alises, Olga, et al., "Prenatal Yoga-Based Interventions May Improve Mental Health during Pregnancy: An Overview of Systematic Reviews with Meta-Analysis." *International journal of environmental research and public health*, vol. 20,2 1556. 14 Jan. 2023.

Waqas, Ahmed, et al., "Prevention of common mental disorders among women in the perinatal period: a critical mixed-methods review and meta-analysis." *Global mental health (Cambridge, England)*, vol. 9 157-172. 23 Mar. 2022.

Warburton, W., et al. "A register study of the impact of stopping third trimester selective serotonin reuptake inhibitor exposure on neonatal health." *Acta psychiatrica Scandinavica*, vol. 121,6 (2010): 471–9.

Weissman, Alicia M, et al. "Pooled analysis of antidepressant levels in lactating mothers, breast milk, and nursing infants." *The American journal of psychiatry*, vol. 161,6 (2004): 1066–78.

Werner, Elizabeth, et al. "Preventing postpartum depression: review and recommendations." *Archives of women's mental health*, vol. 18,1 (2015): 41–60.

Wesseloo, Richard, et al. "Risk of postpartum episodes in women with bipolar disorder after lamotrigine or lithium use during pregnancy: A population-based cohort study." *Journal of affective disorders*, vol. 218 (2017): 394–397.

Wilson, Karen L., et al. "Persistent pulmonary hypertension of the newborn is associated with mode of delivery and not with maternal use of selective serotonin reuptake inhibitors." *American journal of perinatology*, vol. 28,1 (2011): 19–24.

Wisner, K. L., and C. Schaefer. "Psychotropic Drugs," in *Drugs During Pregnancy and Lactation: Treatment Options and Risk Assessment. Academic Press* 2015; 293–339.

Wisner, K. L., et al. "Prevention of recurrent postpartum depression: a randomized clinical trial." *The Journal of clinical psychiatry*, vol. 62,2 (2001): 82–6.

Wisner, Katherine L., et al. "Major depression and antidepressant treatment: impact on pregnancy and neonatal outcomes." *The American journal of psychiatry*, vol. 166,5 (2009): 557–66.

Wisner, Katherine L., et al. "Onset timing, thoughts of self-harm, and diagnoses in postpartum women with screen-positive depression findings." *JAMA psychiatry*, vol. 70,5 (2013): 490–8.

Wisner, Katherine L., et al. "Timing of depression recurrence in the first year after birth." *Journal of affective disorders*, vol. 78,3 (2004): 249–52.

Yamamoto-Sasaki, Madoka, et al. "Association between antidepressant use during pregnancy and autism spectrum disorder in children: a retrospective cohort study based on Japanese claims data." *Maternal health, neonatology and perinatology*, vol. 5 1. 10 Jan. 2019.

Yan, Jing, et al. "Association between Duration of Folic Acid Supplementation during Pregnancy and Risk of Postpartum Depression." *Nutrients*, vol. 9,11 1206. 2 Nov. 2017.

Yonkers, K., et al. "Management of Bipolar Disorder During Pregnancy The Postpartum Period." *Focus* 2005; 3:266–279.

Yonkers, Kimberly A., et al. "The management of depression during pregnancy: a report from the American Psychiatric Association and the American College of Obstetricians and Gynecologists." *General hospital psychiatry*, vol. 31,5 (2009): 403–13.

Young, Sharon M., et al. "Placentophagy's effects on mood, bonding, and fatigue: A pilot trial, part 2." *Women and birth: journal of the Australian College of Midwives*, vol. 31,4 (2018): e258–e271.

Yu, Hang, et al. "Perinatal Depression and Risk of Suicidal Behavior." *JAMA network open*, vol. 7,1 e2350897. 2 Jan. 2024.

Zepeda, Rossana C., et al., "St. John's Wort usage in treating of perinatal depression." *Frontiers in behavioral neuroscience,* vol. 16 1066459. 5 Jan. 2023.

Zhang, Mi-Mi, et al. "The efficacy and safety of omega-3 fatty acids on depressive symptoms in perinatal women: a meta-analysis of randomized placebo-controlled trials." *Translational psychiatry,* vol. 10,1 193. 17 Jun. 2020.

Zhang, Sheng, et al. "The role of gut microbiota in the pathogenesis and treatment of postpartum depression." *Annals of general psychiatry,* vol. 22,1 36. 27 Sep. 2023.

Zimmermann, Martha, et al. "Can psychological interventions prevent or reduce risk for perinatal anxiety disorders? A systematic review and meta-analysis." *General hospital psychiatry,* vol. 84 (2023): 203–214.

Appendix

Terminology

attention deficit/hyperactivity disorder (ADHD)—ADHD is usually a lifelong mental health disorder seen in children and adults. Symptoms include difficulty focusing, with hyperactive and impulsive behavior that can cause difficulties in relationships and work performance.

bipolar disorder—Also known as manic depression, bipolar disorder is characterized by mood swings from manic (see "mania") to depressed. Many researchers believe there is a strong genetic component to this illness. Bipolar disorder occurs on a spectrum of severity. Bipolar I includes repeated episodes of mania and depression. Bipolar II is characterized by recurrent periods of hypomania and depression. Manic episodes can include hallucinations and delusions, which create a medical emergency. Hypomanic swings can include trouble sleeping, irritability, agitation/anxiety, and difficulty concentrating. Often people are considered "moody." Often there is a history of a family member (who may never have been diagnosed) with bipolar disorder.

cognitive behavioral therapy (CBT)—Cognitive behavioral therapy has been well researched and shown to be a very effective form of psychotherapy for perinatal issues.

With CBT, the therapist takes an active role in the therapy process and provides a clear structure and focus to treatment. Cognitive therapy teaches the client how certain thought patterns, beliefs, and behaviors create symptoms such as depression, anxiety, or anger. The therapist works with the client to help develop new positive ways of thinking and acting. CBT encourages and supports the client in creating specific, practical goals, and techniques to achieve them. The focus is on creating new skills.

complementary and alternative medicine (CAM)—These treatments cover a wide variety of therapies. Complementary treatments are used *in addition to* the main treatment as enhancements. Alternative treatments are used *instead of* medication.

cortisol—Called the "stress hormone," cortisol is a hormone released by the adrenal glands during anxious or agitated states.

delusion—This is a false belief. A person may fear being chased or spied on or think she/he is someone other than herself/himself. Often there is religious content to the thoughts.

depression—A common disorder characterized by sad mood, irritability, sleep and appetite disturbances, loss of pleasure, fatigue, and hopelessness. Depression can be caused by a variety of factors, including biochemical, emotional, and psychological.

electroconvulsive therapy (ECT)—A medical procedure used to treat severe depression, bipolar disorder, and psychosis, including during pregnancy, ECT is done under anesthesia 2 or 3 times a week for 6–12 sessions. It can provide rapid improvement in symptoms. Side effects may include memory loss, muscle aches, and soreness.

etiology—The cause or origin of a disease or illness.

hallucination—Something a person sees (visual hallucination) or hears (auditory hallucination) that others do not. Hallucinations often have religious overtones, for example, hearing the voice of God or Satan. These hallucinations often include commands, telling the person they should do certain things.

hypomania—Sometimes confused with the normal joy and excitation of having a new baby, hypomanic symptoms include increased goal-directed activity, being overly talkative, racing thoughts, decreased need for sleep, distractibility, and irritability. There is no significant difficulty with functioning, but hypomania is associated with significant depression later in the postpartum period.

insomnia—Inability to sleep. This can be trouble falling or staying asleep.

interpersonal psychotherapy (IPT)—IPT is a brief and highly structured psychotherapy that addresses interpersonal issues. This model of therapy has been shown to be effective for prenatal and postpartum mood and anxiety disorders.

IPT helps the client solve problems, for instance, disagreements, feeling isolated, adjusting to new roles, or grief following a loss. The therapist works from a collaborative framework.

Low Blue Lights—Televisions, computers, and home light bulbs all contain blue light rays. The blue light tells your brain not to produce melatonin, a hormone that helps your body sleep. Sleep is improved when you increase your level of melatonin. You can buy special glasses or light bulbs that filter out blue light (so you can still watch TV or be on your computer). We recommend LowBlueLights.com.

mania—A symptom of bipolar disorder (see above) characterized by exaggerated excitement, hyperactivity, and racing, scattered thoughts. A person in a manic state feels an emotional "high" and often does not use good judgment. Speech may be rapid, and a person may feel little need for sleep or food. Thinking is usually confused, and a person may act in sexually, socially, and physically unhealthy ways, for instance, inappropriate sexual behavior or shopping sprees.

mindfulness-based cognitive therapy (MBCT)—This therapy combines the ideas and tools of cognitive therapy with meditative practices and breathing exercises. Mindfulness helps focus awareness on the present moment, calmly and without judgment, while acknowledging feelings, thoughts, and bodily sensations.

mood instability—When moods change rapidly. Mood may swing from happy to sad, for instance.

neurotransmitter—Chemical released by nerve cells that carries information from one cell to another. This type of chemical transmits messages in the brain. Some neurotransmitters are serotonin, norepinephrine, and dopamine.

obsessive-compulsive disorder (OCD)—Occurs in about 1 in 100 people. OCD is associated with a chemical imbalance in the brain. This condition worsens in times of stress. Obsessions are thoughts that occur intrusively (they seem to just appear) and repetitively (over and over again). Even with reassurance, people with obsessions continue to worry or have repetitive thoughts. Compulsions are repetitive actions taken to reduce anxiety produced by the obsession. Compulsions often take the form of cleaning, checking (for instance, the locks on the door or the baby's breathing), or counting (for instance, the number of diapers in the bag). A person may have only obsessions, or obsessions and compulsions.

omega-3 fish oil—Pharmaceutical grade is the purest form of fish oil and contains the highest amount of omega-3 fatty acids of EPA and DHA (the "essential" fatty acids). All products are not the same. Look for a product that has a Certificate of Analysis, is USP (United States Pharmacopeia) approved, or tested for purity by a third party. Be sure to check the amounts of EPA and DHA to ensure you are getting 1000 mg of EPA. We encourage you to make sure you buy fish oil that is caught in a way that protects the ocean's ecosystem. Read the label carefully!

panic disorder—During a panic attack, the person may feel symptoms including intense fear, rapid breathing, sweating, nausea, dizziness, and numbness or tingling. Sufferers often fear having the next panic attack and may develop behaviors to avoid situations they think put them at risk.

perinatal mood or anxiety disorder (PMAD)—A mood disorder (for instance, depression) or anxiety disorder (for example, panic) beginning during pregnancy or during the first year postpartum.

phobia—A persistent, irrational fear of a specific object, activity, or situation. This fear usually leads either to avoidance of the feared object or situation, or to experiencing it with dread. Common phobias include fear of heights, flying in airplanes, small places, and spiders.

postpartum—After a mother gives birth. An illness is considered postpartum if it begins in the first year after birth.

post-traumatic stress disorder (PTSD)—PTSD can occur following life-threatening or injury-producing events such as sexual abuse or assault, or traumatic childbirth. People who suffer from PTSD often experience nightmares and flashbacks, have difficulty sleeping, and feel detached. Symptoms can be severe and significantly impair daily life.

premenstrual dysphoric disorder (PMDD)—A combination of symptoms that appear a week or two before a menstrual period, and go away within a week after the onset of the period. Common symptoms include bloating, cramping, irritability, fatigue, anger, and depression. About 75% of women experience some degree of premenstrual mood symptoms.

prenatal—During pregnancy.

psychoanalysis—A form of psychotherapy that focuses on unconscious factors affecting current relationships and patterns of behavior, traces the factors to their origins, shows how they have changed over time, and helps the client cope with adult life. The client talks and the therapist is primarily a listener. Usually therapy takes place four or five times a week, and can continue for years. This is the kind of therapy that's often shown in movies or on television.

psychosis—An extreme and potentially dangerous mental disturbance that includes losing touch with reality. The psychotic person displays irrational behavior and has hallucinations and delusions. Hospitalization and medication are required. It is now thought most postpartum psychosis is due to bipolar illness. Women with psychosis have a higher rate of suicide and infanticide (killing the infant) as a result.

psychotropic medication—Medication that affects thought processes or feeling states by acting on brain chemistry. Antidepressants and antianxiety medications are included in this category.

relapse—To become ill again, after a period of wellness.

sleep hygiene—A variety of practices that help promote good sleep. Some of these include making sure your bedroom is dark, quiet, and relaxing. Avoid alcohol, caffeine, and tobacco close to bedtime. Turn down bright lights and turn off electronics an hour before bed and use glasses that block blue light. Having pets in the bed can sometimes disrupt sleep.

transcranial magnetic stimulation (TMS)—TMS is a therapy that uses electromagnetic fields to stimulate areas in the brain that may be underactive in people suffering from depression. This therapy is prescribed and administered by a medical doctor, usually a psychiatrist. Patients sit in a special chair (like at the dentist), and a magnetic coil is placed on your head for up to an hour every treatment session. Fully alert during sessions, patients can read or watch TV. Treatment is every day (at least 5 days/week) for 4–6 weeks, usually in an office setting. You are able to drive yourself to and from sessions. The most common side effect noted is headache. Some insurance companies will pay for this treatment.

Healthcare Professionals

Note: Licensure varies from state to state. Also, information about perinatal mood disorders is not a routine part of most training programs. See the section in Chapter 3 on finding a knowledgeable therapist or psychiatrist.

certified midwife (CM)—A CM is an individual educated in the discipline of midwifery, who is certified by the American College of Nurse-Midwives. The CM provides primary healthcare to women, including prenatal care, labor and delivery care, care after birth, gynecological exams, newborn care, assistance with family planning, pre-conception care, menopausal management, and counseling in health maintenance.

certified nurse-midwife (CNM)—A CNM is a licensed healthcare practitioner educated in nursing and midwifery. She provides primary healthcare to women of childbearing age, including prenatal care, labor and delivery care, care after birth, gynecological exams, newborn care, assistance with family planning, pre-pregnancy care, menopausal management, and counseling in health maintenance. CNMs attend over 9% of the births in the United States. Many CNMs are able to prescribe medication.

clinical psychologist—Mental health professionals who have earned a doctoral degree in psychology (either a PhD, PsyD, or EdD). They have received extensive clinical training in research, assessment, and the application of different psychological therapies. Clinical psychologists are concerned with the study, diagnosis, treatment, and prevention of mental and emotional disorders. They are not able to prescribe medication.

doula, birth doula—The word *doula* is derived from a Greek word that translates "woman's servant." The certified birth doula's role is to provide physical and emotional support to women and their partners during labor and birth. Birth doulas do not perform clinical tasks such as vaginal exams or fetal heart rate monitoring. Doulas are not trained to diagnose medical or psychological conditions or give medical advice; rather they help women advocate for their birth preferences. Birth doulas educate women regarding physical and emotional comfort measures for labor, birth, and the immediate postpartum period, including initial breastfeeding.

doula, postpartum—There is a difference between a birth doula and a postpartum doula. Postpartum doulas provide physical, emotional, and educational support for women and partners after the baby comes home. Certified postpartum doulas are infant CPR certified, and trained in lactation support, newborn care, nutrition, and emotional adjustment to parenthood in the first weeks of the baby's life. Postpartum doulas will often offer light housework and meal preparation. For more information about certifying agencies, see the Resources section.

Questions to help you select a doula:

Are you certified?

Are you trained in postpartum depression?

What is your view regarding use of medication for depression?

What are the local resources you can help us with regarding postpartum depression?

endocrinologist—A physician (MD) who specializes in treating problems related to hormones. Endocrinologists frequently treat thyroid problems.

lactation consultant—Trained, often certified, specialist who provides support and education about the process of breastfeeding. A lactation consultant can provide help regarding nursing, pumping, bottle feeding, and weaning.

licensed clinical professional counselor (LCPC)—An LCPC is a masters-level mental health professional. LCPCs are not able to prescribe medications.

marriage and family therapist (MFT)—A professional with a master's-level license, MFTs are similar to Licensed Clincial Social Workers and Licensed Professional Counselors. They are trained in individual, couple, and family therapy. None are able to prescribe medication.

midwives, other (see "certified midwife" and "certified nurse-midwife")—Some women practice midwifery without a license. Be sure to ask about training and licensure.

perinatal mental health certified (PMH-C)—PMHs are mental health practitioners, allied professionals (such as doulas and lactation consultants), and prescribers can become certified in perinatal mental health. (See postpartum.net to find a certified provider or for more information about becoming certified.)

physician assistant—PAs are certified medical professionals who diagnose illness, develop and manage treatment plans, prescribe medications, and often serve as patients' principal healthcare providers. PAs can have specialty certification in psychiatry. Most are required to work under the supervision of an M.D. or D.O.

psychiatric nurse (APRN)—Registered nurses who seek additional education and obtain a master's or doctoral degree can become advanced practice registered nurses in a specialty (APRNs). They provide the full range of psychiatric care services to individuals, families, groups, and communities, and in most states they have the authority to prescribe medications. APRNs are qualified to practice independently.

psychiatric social worker—These mental health professionals have earned the MSW (master's degree) in social work) degree and are trained to be sensitive to the impact of environmental factors on mental disorders. LCSW designates licensed clinical social worker. These professionals cannot prescribe medication.

psychiatrist—These mental health professionals have earned the MD (medical doctor) degree. Advanced training focuses on psychiatric diagnosis, psychopharmacology (medication management of mental health issues), and psychotherapy. These physicians are the experts in prescribing psychotropic medications.

psychotherapist—A person who practices psychotherapy: either a clinical psychologist, psychiatrist, professional counselor, social worker, or other mental health professional. Only a medical doctor, clinical nurse specialist, physician assistant, and in some states a psychologist, can prescribe medication.

Endorsements and Awards

Beyond the Blues is a recommended resource by many professionals, organizations, agencies, and educational institutions including:

Brooke Shields, actress and author on Postpartum Depression

Childbirth and Postpartum Professional Association (CAPPA)

Durham Regional Health Department of Canada

First 5 Butte County, California

International Childbirth Education Association. (ICEA)

Michigan Spectrum Health

New York State Department of Health

Pine Rest Christian Mental Health Services

Postpartum Support International (PSI)

Rex Health Center, University of North Carolina

United States Department of Health and Human Services

U.S. Navy

Awards include:

iParenting Media Award

Gold Award, National Parenting Publications

Bronze Award, National Health Information

Seminars, Training, Workshops, and Consultation

Drs. Bennett and Indman offer consultation, lectures, and training on perinatal illness to a wide variety of professionals and organizations. Sample topics include:

- Assessment, diagnosis, and prevention
- Psychotherapy models and techniques
- The latest research in perinatal psychopharmacology
- Consequences of untreated illness
- Resources to help suffering families

They tailor their presentations to fit the particular needs and interests of the participants. Working individually or as a team, they can provide any type of program at your facility, from a brief talk to a comprehensive two-day seminar. Please contact them directly for scheduling and fee information.

Contact Shoshana Bennett or Pec Indman directly:

Shoshana S. Bennett, PhD, PMH-C
DrShosh.com

Pec Indman, PA, EdD, MFT, PMH-C
pecfish@gmail.com

About the Authors

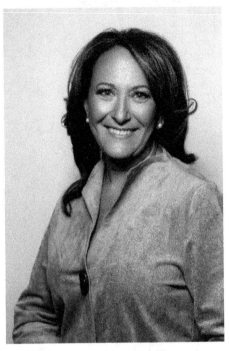

SHOSHANA BENNETT, PhD, PMH-C ("Dr. Shosh"), the mother of Elana and Aaron, founded Postpartum Assistance for Mothers in 1987 after her second experience with two life-threatening postpartum depressions. She is the author of *Children of the Depressed, Pregnant on Prozac* and *Postpartum Depression for Dummies.* National TV shows feature Dr. Shosh as the postpartum expert, and news stations consult her. She's interviewed regularly on national radio and has been quoted in dozens of newspapers and magazines. She is a past president of Postpartum Support International, noted guest lecturer, keynote speaker, creator of the first PPD app, an Executive Producer of the film *Dark Side of The Full Moon,* and Co-Founder of the Postpartum Action Institute. She earned three teaching credentials, two master's degrees, a PhD, and is licensed as a clinical psychologist.

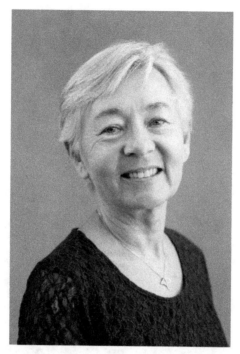

PEC INDMAN, PA, EdD, MFT, PMH-C has a doctorate in counseling and a master's degree in health psychology. She is a retired marriage and family therapist and nationally certified in Perinatal Mental Health. Her training as a physician assistant in family practice was at Johns Hopkins University. Dr. Indman is a Past Chair of Education and Training for Postpartum Support International, and serves on the PSI Advisory Council. She develops curriculum and is a trainer for Postpartum Support International. Dr. Indman has been interviewed on national radio and television, for magazines, newspapers, and videos. Lecturing for a wide variety of audiences nationally and internationally, Dr. Indman has served as an expert advisor for federal and local programs as well as a reviewer for several women's mental health journals and programs. She is an avid scuba diver and underwater photographer.

Index

Abilify 109

acupuncture 15, 99,

alcohol 50, 75, 89, 92, 100, 156

alprazolam 104, 113

alternative therapies and treatments 32, 96, 97, 100

Ambien 111

amitriptyline 111

antianxiety medications 104, 113, 115

antidepressants 47–50, 103–105, 111

aripiprazole 109

Ativan 104, 113

"atypical" antipsychotics 108, 109, 114, 117

attention deficit/hyperactivity disorder (ADHD) 105, 151

autism 92, 105, 107

"Baby Blues" 18, 66

Benadryl 111

benzodiazepine 104–105

bipolar disorder 13, 14, 29, 30, 49, 74, 78, 81, 83, 96, 97, 108–110, 114, 116, 151

breastfeeding/breast milk 30, 34, 39, 44–46, 49-50, 77, 79, 81, 85–86, 90, 98, 100, 108, 103, 113, 114–115

brexanolone 104, 105

cannabis 74, 99

carbamazepine 102, 110, 116

clonazepam 104

cognitive behavioral therapy (CBT) 23, 35, 95, 111, 151

cognitive behavioral therapy with exposure and response prevention (CBT with ERP) 23

cognitive behavioral therapy for insomnia (CBT-I) 111

complementary and alternative medicine CAM) 96–98, 115–118, 152

cortisol 152

COVID-19 12, 35

delusion 26, 80, 152

Depakote 102, 110, 116

Depo-Provera 112

depression, perinatal 11, 12, 31, 38, 55, 56, 93, 152

Deseryl 111

diazepam 104

diphendramamine 111

doulas 37, 83–84, 158-159

doxylamine 111

Edinburgh Postnatal Depression Screening (EPDS) 69, 72, 76–77

Elavil 111

electroconvulsive therapy (ECT) 109, 114, 117, 152

estrogen 112

etiology 152

eye movement desensitization and reprocessing (EMDR) 95

fathers, risk factors 54

fathers, depression 90

folic acid 93, 110

Haldol 108

haloperidol 108

hallucinations 80, 152

herbs 50, 74, 75, 100–101

hormone therapy 112

hypomania 29, 96, 153

infanticide 13, 26

insomnia 5, 74, 79, 153

insurance 34, 157

interpersonal psychotherapy (IPT) 35, 92, 95, 153

Klonopin 104

Lamictal 110, 116

lamotrigine 49, 110, 116

light therapy 97

lithium 110, 116

lorazepam 104, 113

Low Blue Lights 153

mania 29, 96, 153

major depressive disorder (MDD) 16

marijuana 74–75, 89, 99–100

massage 25, 43, 90, 97

mindfulness-based cognitive therapy (MBCT) 93, 154

miscarriage 20, 32, 50, 103–104, 105, 109

mood stabilizers 109–110, 114

neurotransmitter 154

obsessive-compulsive disorder (OCD) 13–14, 54, 78–79, 100–101, 109, 113, 154

olanzapine 109

omega-3 fatty acids 98, 154

panic disorder 13, 24–25, 155

paroxetine 106

Patient Health Questionnaire-9 (PHQ-9) 72–80, 84, 86

Paxil 106

perinatal loss 11, 20, 32, 94

perinatal mood and anxiety disorder (PMAD) 11, 12, 15, 36, 38, 39, 40, 69, 74, 77, 79, 83, 84–86, 92, 94, 96, 102–103, 155

phenytoin 49

phobia 155

placental encapsulation 101

postpartum 155

Postpartum Depression Screening Scale (PDSS) 76

post-traumatic stress disorder (PTSD) 13, 27–28, 155

premenstrual dysphoric mood disorder (PMDD) 20, 25, 155

premenstrual syndrome (PMS) 20, 75

prevention 92–94, 96, 98, 117

progesterone 112

psychosis 13, 26–27, 79, 80, 81, 83, 109, 114–115, 117, 118, 155

quetiapine 109

risk assessment

    Pre-pregnancy and Pregnancy/Prenatal 73–75

    Postpartum 76–80

St. John's wort 96, 100–101

SAMe 96

Seroquel 109

sleep 17, 18, 39–41, 54, 57, 66, 76, 78, 94, 97–98, 110–111, 113, 115, 156

suicide 12, 23, 27, 69

Tegretol 102, 110, 116

therapist, finding 34–35

thyroid/thyroiditis 17, 20, 24, 51, 77, 79, 111–112, 159

transcranial magnetic stimulation (TMS) 21, 98, 156

trazadone 111

triggers, avoidance of potential 28

Unisom 111

Valium 104

valproate 49

valproic acid 102, 110, 116

weaning baby 79, 85–86,159

Xanax 104, 113

zolpidem 111

Zulresso 108

zuranolone 108, 117

Zurzuvae 108, 121

Zyprexa 109

HISTRIA
BOOKS

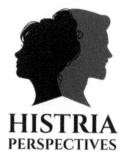

HISTRIA PERSPECTIVES

HISTRIA PERSPECTIVES
BOOKS TO CHALLENGE AND ENLIGHTEN

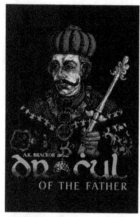

A.K. BRACKOB

DRĂCUL OF THE FATHER

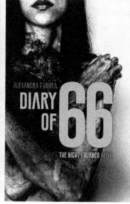

ALEXANDRA FURNEA

DIARY OF 66

THE NIGHT I BURNED ALIVE

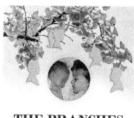

THE BRANCHES *we* **CHERISH**

AN OPEN ADOPTION MEMOIR

LINDA R. SEXTON

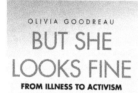

OLIVIA GOODREAU

BUT SHE LOOKS FINE

FROM ILLNESS TO ACTIVISM

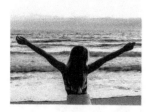

THE SILVER BULLET SOLUTION

IS IT TIME TO END THE WAR ON DRUGS?

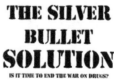

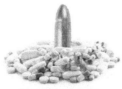

JAMES E. GIERACH

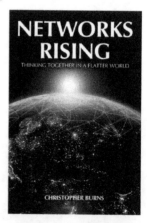

NETWORKS RISING

THINKING TOGETHER IN A FLATTER WORLD

CHRISTOPHER BURNS

FOR THESE AND OTHER GREAT BOOKS VISIT
HISTRIABOOKS.COM